Handbook of Acupuncture
in the Treatment of
Nervous System Disorders

Biographical details

Lü Shaojie is Chief Physician and Director of the Acupuncture Department, Xiangyang Hospital, Henan Province. He was born in 1956 to a family which had practised traditional Chinese medicine for generations. He studied under his father and the direct supervision of Dr. Cheng Xiangsheng, Professor of the Xiangfan Medical School, subsequently graduating from Hubei College of Traditional Chinese Medicine with a degree in Chinese Medicine. He then became a doctor in the Acupuncture Department of Xiangyang Hospital. Now with more than 20 years of clinical experience, Doctor Lü has undertaken much clinical research in TCM, especially in relation to treatment of the sequelae of cardiovascular diseases, spondylosis and pain. He has published a number of books including *Acupuncture in the Treatment of Nervous Diseases* and *Acupuncture in the Treatment of Orthopaedic Diseases*.

Mao Shuzhang, now retired, was Professor of Microbiology at Peking Union Hospital. He has translated a number of books on Western medicine and TCM and is a key translator of the Journal of Traditional Chinese Medicine published by the Academy of Traditional Chinese Medicine.

Robert J Dickie, FRCGP, DRCOG, BMedBiol graduated from Aberdeen University in 1978. After lecturing in pathology for some years, Dr. Dickie then underwent training to become a General Practitioner. Since 1985, he has been a full-time GP on the Isle of Lewis, with particular interests in dermatology and forensic medicine. For many years he has practised homeopathy and acupuncture and offers these services to patients in his NHS practice. He is also involved in training medical undergraduates and postgraduates both in the UK and overseas.

Handbook of Acupuncture

in the Treatment of

Nervous System Disorders

Lü Shaojie

Chief Physician and Director, Acupuncture Department
Xiangyang Hospital, Henan

Translated by

Mao Shuzhang

Professor of Microbiology at Peking Union Hospital

Consultant medical editor

Robert J Dickie

FRCGP, DRCOG, BMedBiol

Donica Publishing Ltd

Note

Medical knowledge is constantly changing. As new information becomes available, changes in treatment, procedures, equipment and the use of drugs become necessary. The editors/authors/contributors and the publishers have, as far as it is possible, taken care to ensure that the information given in this text is accurate and up to date. However, readers are strongly advised to confirm that the information, especially with regard to drug usage, complies with the latest legislation and standards of practice.

Although every effort has been made to indicate appropriate precautions with regard to acupuncture treatment, neither the publishers nor the author can accept responsibility for any treatment advice or information offered, neither will they be liable for any loss or damage of any nature occasioned to or suffered by any person acting or refraining from acting as a result of reliance on the material contained in this publication.

First published 2002

ISBN 1 901149 01 3

British Library Cataloguing in Publication Data
A catalogue record for this book is available from the British Library

Commissioning editor Yanping Li
Managing editor Rodger Watts
Illustrator Maggie Pang

Typeset by Aarontype Ltd.
Printed in the UK by CPI.
The publisher's policy is to use paper manufactured from sustainable forests.

Contents

Chapter 3 Conditions of the spinal nerves

Chapter 4 Other disorders

Editor's foreword

Acupuncture therapy has developed rapidly in the West during the past 30 years and has now become established as a widely accepted treatment method in a variety of contexts. However, the difficulties faced by Western acupuncturists in studying original Chinese-language texts have restricted access to the wealth of experience gained over the centuries by doctors in China, the home of acupuncture.

A practical book on the use of acupuncture in the treatment of disorders of the nervous system is a rarity in the English language. One of the problems in treating this type of disorder is that damage to neural tissue may be so advanced as to be irreversible. There may be some recovery of function as time goes on, partly by temporarily damaged pathways being restored to health, or otherwise by alternative neural pathways taking over the impaired functions. Although research findings have indicated that acupuncture exerts various effects upon the nervous system, the precise mechanisms are not yet fully understood.

Therefore, one of my main concerns in editing this book, which adopts an integrated Chinese-Western approach to the assessment and treatment of a range of nervous system disorders, was to ensure as far as possible that no unsustainable claims were made about the efficacy of acupuncture treatment. In years to come, rigorous evaluation of the techniques may bring further refinements in this context. The treatment methods and techniques described in this book are based on the author's clinical experience over many years and as such offer a valuable insight into the use of acupuncture in treating disorders of the nervous system. The book therefore suggests ways in which acupuncture can be used to alleviate, improve or otherwise treat these disorders and indicates, where appropriate, how acupuncture can form an integral part of a broader treatment scenario.

In editing this book, some differences could be discerned in the definitions of clinical syndromes as a result of occasional variations in circumstances between China and the West. In these and other instances, notably in terms of examination techniques, it was necessary to adapt the text in places to harmonize the clinical features and to conform to standard Western clinical practice.

The long-established tradition of acupuncture in China means that patients there are generally more aware of the types of treatment involved and are possibly more tolerant of the techniques utilized than many patients in the West. As a result, I deemed it necessary to add notes at certain points so that the acupuncturist can advise the patient what to expect in terms of needling sensation and the length and anticipated benefits of acupuncture therapy. Similarly I inserted reminders about important anatomical structures which may be encountered during acupuncture treatment in order to ensure that the procedures remain safe at all times. These various amendments to the original text have been made in consultation with the author.

As the editor of this book, it is my hope that it will be of benefit to fellow practitioners in helping them to treat a variety of disorders of the nervous system, achieve a better understanding of the advantages of acupuncture for these conditions, and offer an effective and safe therapy to their patients. I am grateful to the author for allowing me the opportunity to be involved in this project.

Stornoway
October 2001

Author's foreword

Acupuncture is an indispensable part of traditional Chinese medicine and has a history of over four thousand years. It has developed very rapidly in the last 50 years in China and continues to be used extensively in clinical practice. According to reports appearing in specialist medical journals in China, a significant proportion of the patients attending acupuncture clinics for treatment are affected by neurological disorders. In my experience, acupuncture treatment is particularly applicable to the treatment of nervous system disorders and achieves good results for a number of conditions. Many of these conditions cannot be satisfactorily treated by drugs due to the large number of side effects and the high cost of treatment. Acupuncture treatment is inexpensive, has no side effects and produces highly acceptable results.

I began to practise acupuncture in 1971. After treating thousands of patients and also experimenting with techniques on my own body, I have been able to draw up a systematic analysis of the practical use of acupuncture in the treatment of disorders of the nervous system, partly based on assessment by modern medical diagnostic methods.

In writing this book, I made a careful study of the writings of the great doctors throughout history and drew on the experience of my teachers. Combining this with a modern and realistic approach to the subject, I investigated each disorder and acupuncture point, consulting a variety of sources of clinical material and data. It is my sincere hope that this book will offer readers a new perspective on the treatment of disorders of the nervous system, thus enabling them to improve the effectiveness of the treatment of patients.

This book could not have been written without the constant support and encouragement of Liu Yunzhen and Wei Jiarang, current and former presidents of Xiangyang Hospital, and my wife, Zhou Yucui. I am deeply indebted to them.

Xiangyang
April 2001

Introduction

This practical handbook presents the author's unique clinical experience in the assessment and acupuncture treatment of 57 disorders related to the nervous system and also provides valuable clinical notes offering an insight into the treatment involved.

As the first work of its kind in the English language, this groundbreaking volume is intended for doctors and other health professionals whose main training is in Western medicine, but who also apply acupuncture as a complement or supplement to Western treatment methods. It can likewise be used by doctors and health professionals who have an interest in discovering the benefits of acupuncture in the treatment of disorders related to the nervous system, but who do not practise such therapy themselves; in other words, they can consult this book to decide whether and when to refer a patient for acupuncture treatment for a nervous system disorder, can appreciate the likely results of such treatment, and can take this into account if and when further treatment using Western medical methods is required to improve the condition or complete a cure. In general, all acupuncturists will be able to benefit from study of the clinical symptoms and manifestations in order to use the treatment techniques and point selection discussed for each disorder.

In the West, the growing library of texts in English has provided instruction on acupuncture, diagnostics, pattern differentiation and treatment strategies, but a consistent corpus of specialist acupuncture texts in English has yet to be developed. The author therefore offers this book as a contribution towards building up such a group of works by illustrating how acupuncture functions in a specialist area.

Acupuncture is used widely in China for treating nervous system disorders, especially in relation to cerebrovascular diseases and their sequelae. Wide-ranging research has been carried out both in China and the West into why or how a certain effect can be achieved after stimulation of certain acupuncture points (acupoints). Although more time is required for researchers to formulate a full evidence basis explaining the relationship between acupuncture and the nervous system, clinical findings have indicated that they are indeed related in one way or another.

This book is based on the author's experiences in treating patients with disorders of the nervous system and is therefore a practical book using techniques that the author has perfected over the years. It does not systematically assert that acupuncture always works better than other treatments. The degree of effectiveness of acupuncture in the treatment of disorders of the nervous system depends on a number of factors, such as the length and severity of the disorder and the extent of reversibility, the degree of damage or degeneration already sustained by the affected area of the nervous system, the patient's general condition and accompanying symptoms, the stage at which the patient comes to the acupuncturist for treatment, the type and extent of treatment (including treatment by Western medical techniques) already given, and the patient's willingness to co-operate in the additional treatments suggested to complement acupuncture. Accuracy of location of the relevant acupoints, frequency of treatment and appropriate depth of needling are further keys to success. In addition, acupuncture is used to aid recovery from surgical treatment of some of the nervous system disorders discussed in this book. In the author's experience, acupuncture also has a significant role to play in this respect.

Interest in acupuncture in the West has increased rapidly in the past 30 years. When Western doctors first heard of acupuncture it was greeted with a certain degree of scepticism. Over the succeeding decades, the scientific basis of acupuncture has become accepted and its applicability within the context of conventional Western medicine has been established. In the UK, many doctors now practise acupuncture both in primary care and (to a lesser extent) in secondary care settings. Its value in the management of pain has become widely accepted and it is presently offered as a powerful and effective therapy. However, it is fair to say that the use of acupuncture for disorders of the nervous system has yet to achieve such general acceptance, mainly through a lack of appropriate texts and instructions for its application. It is hoped that this book will make a significant contribution to expanding the use of acupuncture techniques in this area.

One possible reason for the slower acceptance of acupuncture in treating these disorders is the difficulty for doctors trained in Western medicine to adapt to a different philosophy of the origin of disease and its treatment by acupuncture as found in traditional Chinese medicine (TCM). It is therefore instructive to note that traditional medicine nowadays in China is tending towards the adoption of a pragmatic approach to the treatment of most types of diseases and disorders. This means that many of the more recent generations of doctors practise a type of medicine that can be considered as a synthesis of Western and Chinese medicine. In this context, it appears that a proportion of the traditional diagnostic methods that were part and parcel of TCM are being neglected in favour of a more Western approach to diagnosis. Many of the older generation of doctors in China do not support this trend, which has also met stiff opposition among TCM practitioners in the West.

Nevertheless, certain aspects of the present situation in the health sector in China tend to suggest that it is unlikely that this trend towards integrating Western and Chinese medicine will be reversed in the near future. In the first place, TCM and Western medicine are seen as two sides of the same coin in China. All doctors undergo the same basic training in medicine, subsequently specializing in TCM or Western medicine. As a result of their thorough and complete medical training, acupuncturists in China are schooled in the use of techniques that require expert guidance that is possibly harder to find in the West at the 'grass-roots' level.

Secondly, nearly all doctors in China work in hospitals or in clinics within hospitals. This enables greater specialization even at the GP-equivalent level, but also results in a need to see large numbers of patients every day. It is this as much as anything that has caused a shift away from the more time-consuming TCM diagnosis to Western techniques. The greater availability of more expensive medical equipment has also favoured this movement.

However, even where these two factors have resulted in greater attention being paid to Western diagnostic techniques, many doctors and patients still prefer to rely on TCM for the provision of remedies. The clinic set-up and the accessibility of medical care mean that patients will frequently see their doctor on a daily basis until their condition is cured. In addition, the thorough grounding all doctors receive in medical theory and practice allows them to display much greater confidence in needling to a greater depth than is usually the case for Western practitioners of acupuncture. This higher frequency of visits and greater depth of needling is also accepted (and even expected) by patients in China. It does, however, make it more difficult to transfer treatment styles directly from China to the West.

As a result, this book includes certain modifications to the treatment that would be applied in China. These modifications relate principally to the depth of needling. Safety aspects and medicolegal considerations in the UK mean that great caution must be used when needling near to blood vessels, nerves, body cavities and joints, and when practising eye and scalp acupuncture. In situations where there are potential problems with the depths of needling used in TCM, the depth has been reduced to minimize danger whilst at the same time maintaining clinical efficacy. Practitioners wishing to perform the techniques described in this book must follow safe clinical practice at all times: this includes employing single-use disposable needles and minimizing the risk of introducing infection from the skin surface.

In this book, the frequency of treatment remains at the level at which it would be practised in China. Clearly, there is a variety of reasons impeding many patients in the West from attending the clinic on a daily basis. In such cases, treatment will take longer to have an effect than if acupuncture is carried out every day.

In a number of instances, acupuncture treatment needs to be supplemented by other therapies, notably acupoint injections and exercise. It should be noted in the UK context that injection of substances at acupuncture points can only be carried out by health professionals specifically authorized by their qualifications to do so. This would not normally include TCM acupuncturists, unless they have the necessary medical qualifications for administering injections.

Appropriate exercises are often an invaluable aid to completing a successful course of acupuncture treatment. This is indicated in the text where appropriate. Practitioners should always encourage patients to take a responsible attitude to their health and perform the course of exercises suggested.

This book is divided into four chapters; the first three chapters relate to specific parts of the body (cranial nerve disorders, cerebral disorders and conditions of the spinal nerves), whereas the fourth chapter covers a variety of other nervous system disorders. Each condition or disorder starts with a description of its symptoms and clinical manifestations. The descriptions of clinical conditions, including the causative factors for these conditions, may vary a little from those in Western medicine textbooks but will give practitioners an insight into the way in which TCM practitioners in China understand, assess and manage a range of clinical problems. In this context, the investigations suggested by the author have been edited to conform to currently accepted UK practice.

For each condition, the section describing the symptoms and clinical manifestations is followed by a table detailing the acupoints to be selected to treat the condition and the type of needles to be used. For each acupoint, the depth and direction of needle insertion are specified. Unless specifically stated otherwise in the text, needling directions are always given relative to the skin surface. Perpendicular needling therefore indicates insertion at an angle of about 90° to the skin surface and horizontal needling indicates insertion approximately parallel to the skin surface through the subcutaneous tissue after the dermal layer has been penetrated. Other angles of insertion are stated in the text.

Standard acupuncture points are designated by the letter and number coding used in the National Acupuncture Points Standard of the People's Republic of China issued by the State Bureau of Technical Supervision. The locations of non-standard points, in particular those related to tender areas, are described in greater detail. The appendix contains a number of diagrams illustrating the location of all the points used in the book. The practitioner must know how to locate the acupoints accurately and should always take account of the anatomical structures that may be encountered during acupuncture. It is the responsibility of the acupuncturist to ensure that needling will not impinge on or damage important structures such as nerves, joints, blood vessels and internal organs. This is particularly important in treating nervous system disorders, as needling often takes place in the vicinity of the nerve involved.

When needles are inserted, the patient will experience a particular needling sensation at each acupoint; this is indicated for each point in each section. It is good practice to advise the patient of the type of sensation which may be experienced.

Following the table relating to acupoints, there is a description of the method to be followed in administering acupuncture. This indicates the position to be adopted by the patient, the length of time the needles should be retained, the nature and extent of needle manipulation, whether electro-acupuncture is suitable, whether cupping therapy[1] is to be applied when the needles are withdrawn, and the length and frequency of treatment and the interval between repeated courses of treatment.

The clinical notes provide information on the effectiveness of acupuncture treatment for each condition, the optimal time for such treatment, the existence of any contraindications, and additional therapies to support acupuncture.

It is hoped that the treatment principles described in this book will go some way towards promoting understanding of the role that acupuncture can play in treating a variety of nervous system disorders and will contribute to more widespread use of this therapy for these disorders.

---

[1] Cupping therapy is performed by using heat to create a vacuum in specially designed small glass cupping jars, which are then inverted and attached by suction to the skin at the appropriate acupoint(s).

Chapter 1

Cranial nerve disorders

1 OLFACTORY NERVE DISORDERS

Olfactory nerve disorders can be caused by a variety of factors, the most common being the common cold, allergic rhinitis, atrophic rhinitis, nasal polyps, epileptic aura, schizophrenia, hysteria and neurasthenia. Other causes include arrhinencephaly, age-related degeneration of the olfactory organ, meningioma, pituitary tumour, chronic basiarachnoiditis, intracranial hypertension, and primary tumours and metastatic carcinoma of the hippocampal or uncinate gyrus of the temporal lobe.

Clinical manifestations
- anosmia: the sense of smell is markedly decreased or disappears, often accompanied by a decrease in the taste sensation
- hyperosmia: patients are highly sensitive to any kind of odour and feel extremely uncomfortable; this condition is rarely seen
- dysosmia: patients mistake a particular smell for an unpleasant odour; this symptom is often seen in the recovery stage of anosmia. It can also be encountered in head trauma or tabes, and occasionally in pregnant women (possibly related to endocrine factors)
- olfactory hallucination: patients have a hallucination that they can smell an odour, normally bad; this symptom can be seen in cases with epileptic aura, schizophrenia, hysteria and depression

TREATMENT
Acupoints and techniques

Combination of points	Needles used	Insertion technique	Needling sensation
Suliao (DU-25)	No. 32 filiform needle, 1 cun in length	Insert quickly into the subcutaneous tissue, then push along the nasal cartilage towards the nasal bone for 0.3-0.5 cun without rotating the needle shaft; insertion should be quick to avoid pain	Distending and stinging pain at the bridge of the nose

Yingxiang (LI-20, bilateral)	Two no. 30 filiform needles, 1 cun in length	Insert slightly obliquely (at an angle of 15°) towards ala nasi for 0.3-0.5 cun; puncturing at this point is painful, so a similar technique to that employed for DU-25 (above) should be adopted	Distending and stinging pain at the maxillae
Fengchi (GB-20, bilateral)	Two no. 30 filiform needles, 2 cun in length	Insert and push towards the spinal column for 1.0-1.5 cun; as the skin at this location is thick, insertion should be made quickly with the needle then being pushed slowly to the required depth (thus avoiding bending)	Distending pain in the neck and/or pain radiating towards the ipsilateral occiput
Hegu (LI-4, bilateral)	Two no. 30 filiform needles, 1.5 cun in length	Insert towards Yuji (LU-10) for about 1.0 cun	Local distending pain in the thenar muscle

Method

- The patient adopts a sitting position.
- The acupoints are needled, with the needles being retained for 40 minutes; during this period, one session of needle rotation is carried out.
- Acupuncture should be performed once a day for six consecutive days (one course of treatment).
- Recommence the therapy after an interval of three days, if necessary.

Clinical notes
Acupuncture is effective in treating disorders of the olfactory nerve. However, before employing acupuncture, the cause of the disorders should be determined and properly treated first, for example by resection of nasal polyps or elimination of infections or tumours. For common inflammations and hysteria, additional suggestion therapy is very helpful. Acupuncture is very good for the olfactory disorders associated with depression and schizophrenia.

2 RETINAL PERIPHLEBITIS

Retinal periphlebitis (also known as recurring juvenile retinal vitreous haemorrhage) is believed to be related to tuberculosis or focal infections. Delayed hypersensitivity takes place because the tissue of the retinal venous wall is sensitized by tuberculoprotein. However, no active systemic tuberculous focus can be found in most instances. Retinal periphlebitis may also be related to other focal infections or endocrine disorders. The inflammatory damage of the retinal venous wall and its surrounding tissue results in venous thrombosis or rupture of the wall and causes retinal and vitreous haemorrhage.

Clinical manifestations
- often seen in young male patients, with both eyes involved
- at its early stage, muscae volitantes (floaters) and decreased visual acuity can occur due to vitreous haemorrhage; if the haemorrhage is large, visual acuity decreases suddenly and markedly, with only slight residual perception
- exudate or a white perivascular sheath can be seen in the fundus in relation to the involved retinal vein, which is tortuous and deformed
- haemorrhagic spots appear in the adjacent retina
- in severe cases, proliferating retinopathy and secondary retinal detachment may occur

TREATMENT
Acupoints and techniques

Combination of points	Needles used	Insertion technique	Needling sensation
Jingming (BL-1, affected side)	No. 30 filiform needle, 1 cun in length	See below	Distending pain at the eyeball and periocular region
Yiming (EX-HN-14, affected side)	No. 30 filiform needle, 1 cun in length	Insert perpendicularly for 0.5-0.8 cun	Local distending pain

Xinming 1 (affected side): Located at the middle point of the fold posterior to the ear lobe, and 0.5 cun anterosuperior to Yifeng (SJ-17) (see diagram, page 195)	No. 30 filiform needle, 2.5 cun in length	Insert slightly obliquely (at an angle of 15°) and push about 2.0 cun along the lower border of the zygomatic arch towards Tongziliao (GB-1) at the lateral border of the external canthus. The angle of insertion is very important to ensure the desired effect (see diagram, page 199)	Disseminated in the eye
Xinming 2 (affected side): Located at the depression 1 cun superior and 0.5 cun lateral to the lateral end of the eyebrow (see diagram, page 195)	No. 30 filiform needle, 1.5 cun in length	Insert slightly obliquely (at an angle of 15°) and push in the sub-cutaneous plane towards the frontal bone for about 1.0 cun (acupuncture at this point is painful, so insertion should be made quickly and accurately; see diagram, page 199)	Disseminated in the eye

Insertion technique for BL-1: Insert perpendicularly into the orbit for 0.2-0.3 cun after the eyeball is slightly pressed laterally. Insertion and withdrawal should be gentle; no manipulation is performed during insertion. The point should be pressed for a minute or two after withdrawal to avoid lid haemorrhage.

Method
- The patient adopts a sitting position.
- Before BL-1 is needled, the patient should be asked to close the eyes and direct them as far as possible towards the side being needled.

- The acupoints on the affected side are needled, with the needles being retained for one hour; during this period, one session of needle rotation is carried out.
- Acupuncture should be performed once a day for ten consecutive days (one course of treatment).
- Recommence the treatment after an interval of five days, if necessary.

Clinical notes

Although the effectiveness of acupuncture therapy in the treatment of retinal periphlebitis has been demonstrated, close attention must be paid to the accuracy of acupoint location, the angle of insertion and the direction of needle penetration in order to ensure safety of treatment and satisfactory results.

3 OPTIC NEURITIS

Optic neuritis is inflammation of the optic nerve. It is a relatively common problem and may cause acute or chronic visual impairment, sometimes leading to blindness.

The pathogenesis of the disease is various and rather complicated. It can be divided into two categories, local and systemic:
1. local factors: sinusitis, tonsillitis, dental caries, and ocular inflammatory diseases (such as orbital cellulitis, uveitis and chorioretinitis);
2. systemic factors: these include acute infectious diseases (e.g. epidemic meningitis, encephalitis, influenza, parotitis, measles, typhoid fever), chronic infectious diseases (e.g. tuberculosis and syphilis), intoxication (by tobacco, alcohol, methyl alcohol, lead or arsenic), diseases involving demyelination (e.g. optic neuritis and multiple sclerosis), and nutritional and metabolic diseases (e.g. vitamin deficiency, postpartum anaemia, diabetes mellitus, and diseases occurring during pregnancy).

In chronic cases, visual acuity decreases; the prognosis is relatively poor.

Clinical manifestations
Papillitis
- occurs unilaterally or bilaterally
- acute onset, with visual acuity decreasing rapidly
- dragging pain in the periocular region when the involved eye is rotating or is pressed
- central scotoma and concentric constriction of the visual field can be seen on perimetric examination
- the pupillary light reflex seems weak, with the pupil only maintaining constriction for a very short time
- when vision is completely lost, the pupil is dilated and the direct pupillary light reflex disappears

Changes in the ocular fundus
- at the early stage, there may be oedema and congestion of the optic papilla
- the disc margin is blurred; the height of the papilla generally increases by less than 3 dioptres
- the retinal veins may be slightly dilated and tortuous

- the fundus may exhibit mild retinal oedema, flame-shaped haemorrhagic spots and a small amount of exudate around the papilla
- at the advanced stage, optic nerve atrophy occurs

Retrobulbar neuritis
- visual acuity decreases markedly
- central or dumbbell-shaped scotoma occurs in the visual field with peripheral constriction
- dragging pain may be felt during rotation of the involved eye
- at the early stage, the ocular fundus is generally normal or there is slight congestion of the papilla; at the advanced stage, part or all of the papilla can become white (optic atrophy)

TREATMENT
Acupoints and techniques

Combination of points	Needles used	Insertion technique	Needling sensation
Jingming (BL-1, affected side or sides)	No. 30 filiform needle, 1 cun in length	See below	Distending pain at the eyeball and periocular region
Shangming (affected side or sides): Located at the midpoint of the supra-orbital margin on the line between the centre of the arch of the eyebrow and the pupil (see diagram, page 199)	No. 30 filiform needle, 1 cun in length	Insert perpendicularly into the orbit for 0.5-0.8 cun after the eyeball is gently pressed inferiorly (technique and cautions as for BL-1); insert and withdraw slowly	Distending and heavy sensation in the eye
Qiuhou (EX-HN-7, affected side or sides)	No. 30 filiform needle, 1 cun in length	Insert perpendicularly into the orbit for 0.4-0.5 cun after the eyeball is gently pressed superiorly (technique and cautions as for BL-1)	Local distending pain

Fengchi (GB-20, affected side or sides)	No. 30 filiform needle, 2 cun in length	Insert and push towards the spinal column for 1.0-1.3 cun; as the skin at this location is thick, insertion should be made quickly with the needle then being pushed slowly to the required depth (thus avoiding bending)	Distending pain in the neck and/or pain radiating towards the ipsilateral occiput

Insertion technique for BL-1: Insert perpendicularly into the orbit for 0.2-0.3 cun after the eyeball is slightly pressed laterally. Insertion and withdrawal should be gentle; no manipulation is performed during insertion. The point should be pressed for a minute or two after withdrawal to avoid lid haemorrhage.

Method
- The patient adopts a sitting position.
- Before BL-1 is needled, the patient should be asked to close the eyes and direct them as far as possible towards the side being needled.
- Unilateral or bilateral acupoints are selected according to the side or sides affected.
- The acupoints are needled, with the needles being retained for one hour; during this period, one session of gentle needle rotation is carried out.
- Acupuncture should be performed once a day or once every other day for ten sessions (one course of treatment).
- Recommence the treatment after an interval of five days, if necessary.

Clinical notes
Acupuncture is generally effective in the treatment of optic neuritis. During the acute stage, oral medication may also be administered. Subcutaneous haemorrhage may occur in the lid during the acupuncture treatment. If so, acupuncture should be deferred for about five days. If this occurs, apply a cold compress in the first 24 hours, then a hot compress. During absorption of the haematoma, the skin of the lid may turn purplish-blue for a couple of days; this is a common phenomenon.

4 OPTIC ATROPHY

Optic atrophy is characterized by a significant decrease in visual acuity and constriction of the visual field due to degeneration of the optic nerve.

Optic atrophy can be divided into primary and secondary forms. In primary optic atrophy, degeneration is confined to the optic nerve fibres themselves. Retrobulbar optic neuritis is a common cause. Primary optic atrophy may be an early manifestation of tabes, affecting about one-third of patients. Other causes include optic nerve injury following cranial bone fracture, compression by tumours, malnutrition, anaemia and central retinal artery occlusion.

In secondary optic atrophy, there is a proliferation of connective tissue on the optic papilla as well as atrophy of the optic nerve fibres. Secondary optic atrophy is often seen after optic neuritis, optic papillitis, papilloedema, and certain chorioretinal diseases.

Clinical manifestations

- visual acuity decreases gradually or suddenly, with sometimes only slight perception remaining
- visual field constriction, hemianopia, or impairment of colour vision, first for green and then for red; in the later stages, the pupil of the affected eye is dilated

Fundus examination

- in primary optic atrophy, the optic papilla is white, greyish-white or bluish-white, with the papilla slightly smaller than normal; the margin is distinct and regular; the surface microvessels are invisible; the surrounding retina and the retinal blood vessels are normal, although retinal arteries are slightly attenuated
- in secondary optic atrophy, the optic papilla is densely white or greyish-white; the margin is indistinct and irregular; the surface is covered by connective tissue; the cribriform plate and surface microvessels cannot be seen clearly; the retinal arteries are narrow, while the retinal veins are normal or slightly attenuated and tortuous; sometimes there are white sheaths around the retinal vessels close to the papilla

TREATMENT
Acupoints and techniques

Combination of points	Needles used	Insertion technique	Needling sensation
Jingming (BL-1, affected side)	No. 30 filiform needle, 1 cun in length	See below	Distending pain at the eyeball and periocular region
Shangming (affected side): Located at the midpoint of the supra-orbital margin on the line between the centre of the arch of the eyebrow and the pupil (see diagram, page 199)	No. 30 filiform needle, 1 cun in length	Insert perpendicularly into the orbit for 0.5-0.8 cun after the eyeball is gently pressed inferiorly (technique and cautions as for BL-1); insert and withdraw slowly	Distending and heavy sensation in the eye
Taiyang (EX-HN-5, affected side)	No. 30 filiform needle, 1 cun in length	Insert postero-inferiorly at an angle of 75° for 0.5-0.8 cun	Distending sensation disseminating in the retrobulbar region
Yiming (EX-HN-14, affected side)	No. 30 filiform needle, 1 cun in length	Insert perpendicularly for 0.5-0.8 cun	Local distending pain

Insertion technique for BL-1: Insert perpendicularly into the orbit for 0.2-0.3 cun after the eyeball is slightly pressed laterally. Insertion and withdrawal should be gentle; no manipulation is performed during insertion. The point should be pressed for a minute or two after withdrawal to avoid lid haemorrhage.

Method
- The patient adopts a sitting position.
- Before BL-1 is needled, the patient should be asked to close the eyes and direct them as far as possible towards the side being needled.
- The acupoints on the affected side are needled, with the needles being retained for one hour; during this period, one session of needle rotation is carried out.

- Acupuncture should be performed once a day for ten consecutive days (one course of treatment).
- Recommence the treatment after an interval of five days, if necessary.

Clinical notes

Optic atrophy is difficult to cure. The therapeutic effects of the above method are relatively good where cases are treated early; however, the course of treatment is relatively long. Generally, partial or significant visual acuity can be recovered. Although a certain therapeutic effect can be obtained in cases of prolonged duration, the effect is not as good as in cases treated at an early stage.

5 MYOPIA

Myopia (short sight) is a refractive error. The external eye generally has no significant abnormality; the near vision of the eye is good but distant objects are blurred. The pathogenesis of this condition is not clear, but its main manifestation is an increase in the length of the anteroposterior axis of the eyeball. The lengthening of the eyeball axis is closely related to genetic factors, constitution, work and the environment. Sustained use of the eyes or negligence of eye care or health care (prolonged reading, writing or drawing in dimly-lit conditions) are also important predisposing factors. Overusage of accommodation and convergence may cause an increase in intraocular pressure, eventually resulting in lengthening of the ocular axis.

Clinical manifestations
- good near eyesight, but poor distant sight
- no marked abnormality of the external eye
- the higher the degree of myopia, the greater the decrease in distant sight
- in cases with relatively high myopia, patients often narrow their eyes to improve distant vision; this allows external light to pass through the central portion of the cornea only and makes the image formed at the retina clearer (and is analogous to the use of a pinhole during eye examination)
- cases with moderate or high myopia usually originate from muscle fatigue because of a lack of co-ordination between accommodation and convergence
- exotropia (divergent squint) may occur in cases with high myopia or anisometropia
- fundus examination: features such as myopic crescent at the temporal side of the optic papilla, tigroid (or tessellated) retina, retinal degeneration, macular haemorrhage, vitreous opacity, and retinal detachment can be seen in a highly myopic fundus. Fundal changes may aggravate visual impairment and visual field damage

TREATMENT
Acupoints and techniques

Combination of points	Needles used	Insertion technique	Needling sensation
Jingming (BL-1, bilateral)	Two no. 30 filiform needles, 1 cun in length	See below	Distending pain at the eyeball and periocular region
Chengqi (ST-1, bilateral)	Two no. 30 filiform needles, 1.5 cun in length	Insert perpendicularly for 0.5-1.0 cun at each side after the eyeballs have been slightly pressed superiorly	Distending pain in the orbit
Shangming (bilateral): Located at the mid-point of the supra-orbital margin on the line between the centre of the arch of the eyebrow and the pupil (see diagram, page 199)	Two no. 30 filiform needles, 1 cun in length	Insert perpendicularly into the orbit for 0.5-0.8 cun after the eyeball is gently pressed inferiorly (technique and cautions as for BL-1); insert and withdraw slowly	Distending and heavy sensation in the eye
Fengchi (GB-20, bilateral)	Two no. 30 filiform needles, 2 cun in length	Insert and push towards the spinal column for 1.0-1.3 cun; as the skin at this location is thick, insertion should be made quickly with the needle then being pushed slowly to the required depth (thus avoiding bending)	Distending pain in the neck and/or pain radiating towards the ipsilateral occiput

Insertion technique for BL-1: Insert perpendicularly into the orbit for 0.2-0.3 cun after the eyeball is slightly pressed laterally. Insertion and withdrawal should be gentle; no manipulation is performed during insertion. The point should be pressed for a minute or two after withdrawal to avoid lid haemorrhage.

Method
- The patient adopts a sitting position.
- Before BL-1 is needled, the patient should be asked to close the eyes and direct them as far as possible towards the side being needled.
- The acupoints are needled, with the needles being retained for 40 minutes; during this period, one session of gentle needle rotation is carried out.
- Acupuncture should be performed once every other day for ten sessions (one course of treatment).
- Recommence the treatment after an interval of three days, if necessary.

Clinical notes
The therapeutic effects of acupuncture for mild myopia are relatively good, and the visual acuity of the majority of patients with mild myopia (visual acuity over 6/10, or 0.6) can be raised to 6/6, or 1.0, within three courses of treatment. For cases with moderate myopia, some therapeutic effect can be obtained, but the course of treatment will be relatively long; after termination of the therapy, the increase in visual acuity is likely to regress relatively fast, although vision will still be better than before treatment. The therapeutic effect is not satisfactory in cases with high myopia and fundal changes. After treatment, patients should be advised to correct any bad habits in using the eyes; only in this way can the effects of the treatment be consolidated.

6 OCULOMOTOR PARALYSIS

Damage to the oculomotor nerve may be caused by a variety of factors:

- infection or inflammation: this category is often seen and may result from viral infection, periorbital cellulitis, periostitis, rheumatic fever, diphtheria, malnutritional neuritis, cranial basal meningitis often concurrent with otitis media, thrombotic venous sinusitis, syphilis, or tuberculous encephalitis. The primary disease directly involves the oculomotor nerve or its nucleus in the mid-brain;
- myasthenia gravis and myodystrophy: often involves the oculomotor nerve, resulting in paralysis of the nerve;
- trauma: the oculomotor nerve can be compressed or irritated by periorbital bone fracture or haematoma as in cerebral injury, leading to paralysis;
- compression: tumours in the brain, the brain stem, the cervical spinal cord or the neck, and spinobulbar syringomyelia can directly or indirectly involve the oculomotor nerve nucleus in the mid-brain;
- endocrine diseases: dysfunction of the thyroid or pituitary gland.

Clinical manifestations

Clinically, the disease can be divided into two types:

Complete paralysis

- the three cardinal characteristics are flaccid ptosis of the upper lid, exotropia with mild hypotropia (where the affected eye is deviated lower than the unaffected eye), and dilatation of the pupil with disappearance of the light reflex
- because the eyeball is nearly completely covered by the drooping upper lid, the patient may sometimes open the eye a little by contracting the frontal muscle as a compensatory measure to elevate the upper eyelid and occasionally the healthy eye may also have compensatory over-elevation of the upper lid
- the head often deviates to the contralateral side of the involved eye

Incomplete paralysis

- this condition is more common than complete paralysis
- paralysis is mild and involves only one muscle – in most instances, the medial rectus muscle; diagnosis is difficult

TREATMENT
Acupoints and techniques

Combination of points	Needles used	Insertion technique	Needling sensation
Yangbai (GB-14, affected side)	No. 30 filiform needle, 1.5 cun in length	Insert horizontally inferiorly towards and past Yuyao (EX-HN-4); stop at the superior third of the upper eyelid. As this acupoint is close to the frontal bone, insertion should be quick to minimize pain	Distending pain in the forehead and orbit
Cuanzhu (BL-2, affected side) joining Sizhukong (SJ-23)	No. 30 filiform needle, 2 cun in length	Pinch the skin and insert the needle slightly obliquely (at an angle of 15°) at BL-2 for about 0.2 cun and then join SJ-23 horizontally	Distending pain in the orbit
Shangming (affected side): Located at the midpoint of the supra-orbital margin on the line between the centre of the arch of the eyebrow and the pupil (see diagram, page 199)	No. 30 filiform needle, 1 cun in length	Insert perpendicularly into the orbit for 0.5-0.8 cun after the eyeball is gently pressed inferiorly (technique and cautions as for Jingming [BL-1], see section 2); insert and withdraw slowly	Distending and heavy sensation in the eye
Taiyang (EX-HN-5, affected side)	No. 30 filiform needle, 1 cun in length	Insert at an angle of 25° towards the tip of the ear for about 0.3 cun	Distending pain in the temporal region and/or pain radiating to the medial upper part of the eyeball

Method

- The patient adopts a sitting position.
- The acupoints are needled using electro-acupuncture, with the needles being retained for 40 minutes.
- Press the points with a sterilized cotton ball after withdrawal of the needles, thus avoiding haemorrhage.
- Acupuncture should be performed once a day for six consecutive days (one course of treatment).
- Recommence the therapy after an interval of five days, if necessary.

Clinical notes

Oculomotor paralysis is not often encountered. When electro-acupuncture is used for treatment of paralysis not induced by a lesion in the cranial nucleus, the therapeutic effects are relatively satisfactory.

During the period of treatment, the patient should have the involved eye covered to avoid eye disorders or migraine resulting from dilatation of the pupil. After recovery, the patient should be advised to reduce alcohol intake, not to work too late at night and to exercise frequently in order to avoid any recurrence.

In cases with oculomotor paralysis caused by cerebral tumour, intracranial inflammation, craniocerebral injury, and cerebrovascular accident, the primary disease should be relieved first, and the paralysis then treated with acupuncture; the therapeutic effect is also satisfactory. If paralysis recurs, it can be treated as above, again achieving favourable results.

7 TROCHLEAR PARALYSIS

Trochlear paralysis involves paralysis of the superior oblique muscle of the orbit due to inflammation, compression or a lesion of the fourth cranial nerve.

There are two types of pathogenesis:

- intracranial lesions: direct compression on the trochlear nucleus such as a tumour in the brain stem, basal meningitis (often by spread from otitis media), thrombotic cerebral venous sinusitis, syphilis, tuberculous encephalitis, or traction on the trochlear nerve due to intracranial hypertension;
- extracranial lesions: direct or indirect compression on or involvement of the trochlear nerve by viral infections, periorbital cellulitis, periostitis or trauma.

Clinical manifestations
- the involved eyeball is slightly higher than the healthy eye
- diplopia appears when the affected eye looks in any direction other than superolateral gaze
- diplopia makes it difficult for patients to walk downstairs
- when both eyes look vertically upwards, there is a mean separation of $10°-20°$ compared with less than $3°$ normally
- the height of the upper lid of the healthy eye is sometimes lower than that of the involved eye; trochlear paralysis is therefore sometimes misdiagnosed as partial oculomotor paralysis of the healthy eye. This phenomenon is thought to be due to over-relaxation of the superior palpebral levator in the healthy eye

Examination
- significant hypertropia in the affected eye (i.e. the eye is deviated superiorly) when the patient's gaze is towards the superior and contralateral (healthy eye) side
- head-tilt test: the eyes will turn to the opposite direction when the head is tilting. When the superior oblique muscle is paralysed, the affected eye turns superiorly
- to avoid diplopia, patients often tilt their head spontaneously towards the direction of the action of the paralysed muscle. In the diplopia test, the vertical distance between the two images will be largest when the patient fixes the gaze towards the lower contralateral side

TREATMENT
Acupoints and techniques

Combination of points	Needles used	Insertion technique	Needling sensation
Yangbai (GB-14, affected side)	No. 30 filiform needle, 1.5 cun in length	Insert horizontally inferiorly towards and past Yuyao (EX-HN-4); stop at the superior third of the upper eyelid. As this acupoint is close to the frontal bone, insertion should be quick to minimize pain	Distending pain in the forehead and orbit
Taiyang (EX-HN-5, affected side)	No. 30 filiform needle, 2 cun in length	Insert horizontally and push towards Touwei (ST-8) for about 1.4 cun	Distending pain over the lower temporal region and/or pain radiating to the medial upper part of the eyeball
Guangming (GB-37, unaffected side)	No. 30 filiform needle, 2 cun in length	Insert perpendicularly for 1.0-1.5 cun	Pain radiating towards the dorsum of the foot or the heel

Method
- The patient adopts a sitting position.
- The acupoints on the affected side are needled; electro-acupuncture should be used for GB-14 and EX-HN-5.
- The needles are retained for 40 minutes.
- Acupuncture should be performed once a day for six consecutive days (one course of treatment).
- Recommence the therapy after an interval of five days, if necessary.

Clinical notes
The clinical manifestations of trochlear paralysis are relatively mild, so diagnosis is sometimes difficult. Acupuncture is effective in treating simple trochlear paralysis. If the paralysis is due to intracranial inflammation or tumour, the primary disease should be treated first; thereafter, satisfactory therapeutic results can also be obtained. During treatment, the patient should cover the affected eye to avoid diplopia.

8 TRIGEMINAL NEURALGIA

Trigeminal neuralgia (also known as tic douloureux) is a facial pain syndrome of unknown cause that develops in middle to late life. In many instances, it is believed that the traumatic formation of a short circuit between the demyelinated fibres of the sensory root of the trigeminal ganglion and its adjacent motor axons may cause the disorder. Instances of arteriosclerotic change or ectopy of the nutrient artery of the nerve, thickening of the meninges, and compression of the nerve are considered as other aetiological factors.

Causes of the disorder may include lesions of the trigeminal nerve and compression of adjacent tissue accompanied by pathological changes, such as tumours and inflammation or trauma of the ear, nose or teeth.

Clinical manifestations

• often occurs after middle age without marked sex predilection
• sudden pain without predisposing symptoms
• mild stimulation of a key trigger point may elicit excruciating pain; the condition is usually unilateral, often involves the maxillary and mandibular nerves, and seldom involves all three divisions of the nerve simultaneously
• recurrent piercing and lightning-like pain in the region along the nerve, with short episodes of one or two minutes and accompanied by reflex convulsion of facial muscles, facial flushes, conjunctival suffusion, lacrimation, and salivation
• pain abates spontaneously and may not recur for several weeks

TREATMENT
Acupoints and techniques

Combination of points	Needles used	Insertion technique	Needling sensation
Sibai (ST-2, affected side)	No. 30 filiform needle, 1 cun in length	Insert obliquely (at an angle of 45°) along the infra-orbital foramen for 0.3-0.5 cun	Local distending pain

Hegu (LI-4, affected side)	No. 30 filiform needle, 2 cun in length	Insert towards Houxi (SI-3) for 1.0-1.5 cun	Distending pain in the palm
Taiyang (EX-HN-5, affected side)	No. 30 filiform needle, 1.5 cun in length	Insert horizontally and push towards the angle of the mandible for 1.0-1.3 cun, with the posterior part of the zygomatic arch being traversed en route	Local distending pain
Xiaguan (ST-7, affected side)	No. 30 filiform needle, 1.5 cun in length	Insert perpendicularly for 0.5-1.0 cun, taking care to avoid the facial nerve	Local distending pain

Method

- The patient adopts a sitting position.
- During each session, acupuncture is performed in combination with the above points at the two Ahshi points[1] of the local tender area on the face using no. 30 filiform needles, 1 cun in length; insert to a depth of about 0.5 cun.
- The needles are retained for 40 minutes, without rotation during retention or at withdrawal.
- Acupuncture should be performed once a day for ten consecutive days (one course of treatment).
- If the treatment is effective, the next course can be repeated after an interval of about five days.

---

[1] Ahshi points (literally 'ouch' points) are acupuncture points of no fixed location, which are found by eliciting tenderness or pain at the site of greatest sensitivity. They are needled according to the principle that where is pain, there is an acupuncture point.

Addendum: Retention of intradermal needle at the tender point(s)
- Select one or two tender or trigger points in the area of distribution of the trigeminal nerve and insert one or two sterilized skin needles in the centre of the point after routine disinfection of the skin.
- Keep the needle in the subcutaneous tissue for two to three days and protect the needle puncture with an alcohol-steeped cotton ball the size of the external needle shaft ring; the ball is kept in place by an adhesive plaster. If this treatment is effective, repeat the procedure after an interval of one day until a cure is obtained.

Clinical notes

Trigeminal neuralgia is an obstinate condition to treat. As the first choice for non-surgical treatment, acupuncture may be effective in mild cases at an early stage. However, in obstinate cases with frequent daily attacks, acupuncture may only be effective in combination with local corticosteroid injection. Correct selection of indications is the key point for success in using these injections. Because of the high incidence of complications in this type of therapy, the procedure must be performed carefully and accurately. If the therapeutic effects of the above methods are unsatisfactory, they should be halted and the patient referred to a Western medical specialist for consideration of surgical measures such as trigeminal rhizotomy.

For trigeminal neuralgia with a clear underlying cause such as tumour, intracranial hypertension or nosebleed, the first measure is to deal with the primary cause. Thereafter, residual trigeminal neuralgia can be treated by acupuncture, and relatively satisfactory therapeutic effects obtained.

In short, the treatment of this disease is relatively difficult, and recurrence rates are high after initial recovery. Therefore, acupuncture, corticosteroid injection and surgery are only partly helpful in ameliorating the neuralgia.

9 ABDUCENT (LATERAL RECTUS) NERVE PARALYSIS

Abducent paralysis affects the lateral rectus muscle of the eye. It is caused by a variety of factors that affect the abducent nerve directly or indirectly.

The pathogenic causes of abducent paralysis fall into one of the following two categories:
- intracranial diseases which compress or affect the nerve, such as brain tumour, intracranial haematoma, hypertensive cerebral diseases (for example, cerebral haemorrhage or cerebral infarction), intracranial hypertension induced by encephalitis, or meningitis;
- extracranial diseases which directly or indirectly involve the abducent nerve, such as arteriosclerosis of the nutrient artery of the nerve, inflammation in the cavernous sinus or around the internal carotid artery, orbital inflammation, trauma, fracture, or nasopharyngeal carcinoma.

Clinical manifestations
- most commonly seen as a single cranial nerve paralysis
- when the muscle is paralysed, the eyeball on the affected side will be adducted; when the affected eye gazes at a fixed position, marked esotropia (convergent strabismus) will appear in the healthy eye, resulting in diplopia
- in cases of mild paralysis, the patient's head often turns towards the paralysed side or tilts slightly forward as a compensatory mechanism
- bilateral abducent paralysis may occur with intracranial hypertension

TREATMENT
Acupoints and techniques

Combination of points	Needles used	Insertion technique	Needling sensation
Yangbai (GB-14, affected side)	No. 30 filiform needle, 1.5 cun in length	Insert horizontally inferiorly towards and past Yuyao (EX-HN-4); stop at the superior third of the upper eyelid. As this acupoint is close to the frontal bone, insertion should be quick to minimize pain	Distending pain in the forehead and orbit

Cuanzhu (BL-2, affected side), joining Sizhukong (SJ-23)	No. 30 filiform needle, 2 cun in length	Pinch the skin and insert the needle slightly obliquely (at an angle of 15°) at BL-2 for about 0.2 cun and then join SJ-23 horizontally	Distending pain in the orbit
Taiyang (EX-HN-5, affected side)	No. 30 filiform needle, 2 cun in length	Insert horizontally posteriorly towards Shuaigu (GB-8) for 1.0-1.5 cun	Distending pain in the temporal region
Tianzhu (BL-10, affected side)	No. 30 filiform needle, 1 cun in length	Insert perpendicularly for 0.5-0.8 cun	Local distending pain

Method

- Unilateral or bilateral acupoints are selected according to the side or sides affected.
- The patient adopts a sitting position.
- The acupoints are needled using electro-acupuncture, with the needles being retained for 40 minutes.
- Press the points with a sterilized cotton ball after withdrawal of the needles, thus avoiding haemorrhage.
- Acupuncture should be performed once a day for seven consecutive days (one course of treatment).
- Recommence the therapy after an interval of three days, if necessary.

Clinical notes

For simple abducent paralysis caused by inflammation, the therapeutic effects of acupuncture are relatively satisfactory. In cases where the paralysis results from an intracranial lesion, the primary disease should be relieved before performing acupuncture. If the paralysis is caused by cerebral haemorrhage or embolism, acupuncture therapy can be performed simultaneously with treatment of the primary disease by adding treatment at the visual area. During the treatment, the patient can wear a pair of tinted spectacles to avoid overexerting the eye, which would hamper the therapeutic effect.

10 FACIAL TIC

Facial tic is characterized by unilateral or bilateral paroxysmal irregular involuntary spasm of the facial muscles; it is also known as convulsive tic of the facial muscles or facial spasm.

Facial tic is a condition of unclear cause and often occurs when pathological stimulation affects the pathway of the facial nerve. In some cases, it is precipitated by compression from an aneurysm or arteriosclerotic dilation of the branches of the vertebrobasilar artery system, by demyelination after facial neuritis, or by inflammatory lesions or tumours at the pontine angle.

Clinical manifestations
- often occurs in middle-aged female patients with no other symptoms and no history of facial neuritis
- at the early stage, the tic of the orbicularis oculi muscle occurs irregularly, gradually extending to other ipsilateral facial muscles, presenting as a unilateral or bilateral paroxysmal irregular tic of the eyelids and mouth angle. It may persist for several seconds or several minutes and can be aggravated by fatigue or emotional stress; the tic does not occur during sleep
- generally it occurs unilaterally; bilateral involvement is infrequent
- an electromyogram may show muscular fibre and bundle tremor waves

TREATMENT
Acupoints and techniques

Combination of points	Needles used	Insertion technique	Needling sensation
Qianzheng (affected side): Located 0.5 cun anterior to and level with the medial point of the ear lobe (see diagram, page 195)	No. 30 filiform needle, 2 cun in length	Insert slightly obliquely (at an angle of 15°) for about 1.3 cun towards the apex of the nose; in order to avoid injury to the parotid gland and the mandibular vessels, do not puncture too deeply	Local distending pain and heavy sensation

Taiyang (EX-HN-5, affected side)	No. 30 filiform needle, 2 cun in length	Insert horizontally posteriorly towards Shuaigu (GB-8) for 1.0-1.5 cun	Distending pain in the temporal region
Sibai (ST-2, affected side)	No. 30 filiform needle, 1 cun in length	Insert obliquely (at an angle of 45°) along the infra-orbital foramen for 0.3-0.5 cun	Local distending pain
Dicang (ST-4, affected side)	No. 30 filiform needle, 2 cun in length	Insert horizontally to join Jiache (ST-6)	Local distending pain

Method

- The patient adopts a sitting position.
- The acupoints are needled (on one or both sides depending on the location of the facial tic), with the needles being retained for one hour; no needle manipulation takes place.
- Acupuncture should be performed once a day for ten consecutive days (one course of treatment).
- Recommence the treatment after an interval of five days, if necessary.

Clinical notes

A relatively long period of acupuncture treatment is required to obtain a noticeable therapeutic effect in treating facial tic. Mild cases can be cured and the condition of patients with a long history and frequent occurrences of the disorder can be improved. Corticosteroid injection can also be tried in such cases. However, the risk of permanent facial paralysis means that these injections should be performed very carefully on selected patients only. If there is a primary focus, it should be treated first before acupuncture therapy. If acupuncture and injection therapies fail in treating obstinate cases, the patient should be referred to a Western medical specialist for consideration of appropriate surgical measures.

11 FACIAL PARALYSIS (BELL'S PALSY)

Facial paralysis refers to disturbance, impairment or abnormality of function in the region innervated by the extracranial facial nerve (cranial nerve VII), usually due to viral infection. It is also known as facial neuritis or peripheral facial paralysis.

Two factors may participate in the origin of facial paralysis: the lesion itself (for example, ischaemia and oedema due to nutritional impairment of the nerve, and spasm of the nutritional vessels), or involvement or compression by lesions around the nerve (for example, the compression and inflammation of surrounding tissues due to bacterial or viral infections or rheumatism). Periostitis of the stylomastoid foramen can also compress the nerve, leading to impairment of blood circulation and facial paralysis. The main pathological changes are oedema and degeneration; if the condition is prolonged without treatment, the nerve may atrophy.

Clinical manifestations
- may occur at any age; often seen in female patients aged 18-25
- most cases are unilateral, with relatively acute onset
- paralysis of the facial muscles is present on the affected side
- the patient is unable to wrinkle the forehead or contract the eyebrows
- the eyeball rotates upwards and laterally (Bell's sign); when the patient attempts to close the eye, the affected globe remains partially exposed
- the nasolabial groove becomes shallower or disappears, and the angle of the mouth inclines towards the healthy side
- the patient cannot whistle, and food is easily trapped between the teeth and buccal wall on the affected side
- when the lesion is at or distal to the stylomastoid foramen, the only symptom is paralysis of the ipsilateral facial muscles
- when the lesion is in the facial nerve canal between the tympanic cord and stapedius branches, the manifestations are facial paralysis, decrease or disappearance of taste sensation in the anterior two-thirds of the tongue, and impairment of salivary gland secretion
- when the lesion is between the stapedius branch and the geniculate ganglion, hyperacusis is added to the above symptoms

- when the geniculate ganglion is damaged, secretion of the lacrimal gland is diminished or defective and herpes zoster may occur at the external auditory meatus, the lateral side of the auricle and the back of the ear

TREATMENT
Acupoints and techniques

Combination of points	Needles used	Insertion technique	Needling sensation
Taiyang (EX-HN-5, affected side)	Two no. 30 filiform needles, 2 cun in length	Insert one needle horizontally posteriorly towards Shuaigu (GB-8) for 1.0-1.5 cun, and the other horizontally inferiorly towards Jiache (ST-6) for 1.0-1.5 cun	Distending pain in the temporal and buccal regions
Qianzheng (affected side): Located 0.5 cun anterior to and level with the medial point of the ear lobe (see diagram, page 195)	No. 30 filiform needle, 2 cun in length	Insert slightly obliquely (at an angle of 15°) for about 1.3 cun towards the apex of the nose; in order to avoid injury to the parotid gland and the mandibular vessels, do not puncture too deeply	Local distending pain and heavy sensation
Dicang (ST-4, affected side)	No. 30 filiform needle, 2 cun in length	Insert horizontally to join ST-6	Local distending pain

Method

- The patient adopts a sitting position.
- The acupoints are needled using electro-acupuncture, with the needles being retained for one hour.
- Acupuncture should be performed once a day for ten consecutive days (one course of treatment).
- Recommence the treatment after an interval of three days, if necessary.

Clinical notes

The therapeutic effect of electro-acupuncture is particularly satisfactory for simple facial paralysis (if not caused by tumour compression or purulent mastoiditis) and is superior to other therapies. The optimal time to commence acupuncture is within five days of onset of the condition. If the treatment is delayed until more than three and a half months after onset, the therapeutic effects are relatively poor and the course of treatment will be long, but a certain effect can still be achieved. In cases with an underlying cause, this cause should be eliminated first; in the meantime, electro-acupuncture can be applied with satisfactory results.

12 GLOSSOPHARYNGEAL PARALYSIS

Glossopharyngeal paralysis is a progressive paralysis affecting the muscles of the lips, tongue and pharynx and leading to the decrease or loss of sensory functions in the region distributed by the involved nerve.

Simple glossopharyngeal paralysis is rarely seen and often co-exists with damage to other cranial nerves. The main causes are operative division of the nerve, tonsillectomy, and in some cases, compression brought about by tumour or inflammation at the pharynx, larynx or floor of the mouth. Glossopharyngeal paralysis is virtually always accompanied by other cranial nerve damage.

Clinical manifestations
- patients with glossopharyngeal damage suffer sensory impairment; the taste sensation in the posterior third of the tongue is diminished or absent
- general sensations in the upper part of the pharynx are also diminished or lost; this is accompanied by hyporeflexia or areflexia of the pharynx and soft palate
- unilateral areflexia of the pharynx and palate is of pathological significance, but bilateral areflexia without other symptoms has no practical importance because it may also be present in healthy persons
- where the glossopharyngeal nerve is damaged, paralysis of the stylopharyngeus and pharyngopalatine muscles may occur, resulting in prolapse of the soft palate

Examination
- the affected palatine arch is lower than on the healthy side and the uvula is displaced towards the healthy side
- after repetitive phonation and pharyngeal reflex tests, fatigue will cause areflexia to appear on the affected side
- difficulty in swallowing: water may spill from the nostrils, and food and saliva may stagnate in the pharyngeal cavity
- difficulty in phonation: laryngeal phonation is particularly difficult, so the patient speaks with a nasal intonation
- difficulty in elevating the soft palate bilaterally: when resting, the soft palate is relaxed and flaccid, and the pharyngeal reflex is lost

TREATMENT
Acupoints and techniques

Combination of points	Needles used	Insertion technique	Needling sensation
Renying (ST-9, affected side)	No. 30 filiform needle, 1.5 cun in length	Insert towards the spinal column to a depth of 0.5-1.0 cun; care should be taken to avoid the common carotid artery	Local distending pain or distending pain in the neck and throat
Lianquan (RN-23)	No. 30 filiform needle, 1.5 cun in length	Insert towards the root of the tongue for about 1.2 cun	Distending and heavy sensation in the root of the tongue
Neiguan (PC-6, affected side)	No. 30 filiform needle, 1.5 cun in length	Insert perpendicularly towards Waiguan (SJ-5) for 1.0-1.3 cun, taking care to avoid damage to the median nerve	Local distending pain and/or pain radiating to the dorsum of the hand and middle finger
Hegu (LI-4, affected side)	No. 30 filiform needle, 1.5 cun in length	Insert towards Yuji (LU-10) for about 1.0 cun	Local distending pain in the thenar muscle

Method
- The patient adopts a sitting position, with the head tilted backwards.
- Unilateral or bilateral acupoints are selected according to the side or sides affected.
- The acupoints are needled using electro-acupuncture, with the needles being retained for 40 minutes.
- Acupuncture should be performed once a day for six consecutive days (one course of treatment).
- Recommence the treatment after an interval of five days, if necessary.

Clinical notes

The therapeutic effect is extremely satisfactory when electro-acupuncture is applied in the treatment of unilateral glossopharyngeal paralysis. The condition can normally be cured within two courses of treatment. Electro-acupuncture is also effective in treating bilateral glossopharyngeal paralysis. However, most cases are complicated by inflammation in the nasopharynx, trachea or lung. If this is treated adequately during electro-acupuncture, satisfactory results can also be obtained.

13 GLOSSOPHARYNGEAL NEURALGIA

Glossopharyngeal neuralgia manifests as severe paroxysmal pain occurring in the area innervated by the glossopharyngeal nerve and the auditory and pharyngeal branches of the vagus nerve. The characteristics of glossopharyngeal neuralgia are similar to those of trigeminal neuralgia, but it is seen much more rarely.

The aetiology is not clear; possible causes are demyelination or involvement of the nerve due to compression resulting from arachnoiditis or aneurysm or tumours at the cerebellopontine angle, carotid vein foramen, cranial base, nasopharyngeal area and tonsil.

Clinical manifestations
- mostly occurs in patients over 40 years old, with men being more affected than women
- the pain is located at the root of the tongue or the pharyngeal wall around the tonsil, radiating to the nasopharynx or deeper part of the ear and is precipitated by swallowing, speaking, coughing, yawning or other tongue movements
- there are trigger points on the posterior wall of the pharynx, tongue root and tonsillar fossa
- attacks may last from several seconds to one or two minutes, and are sometimes accompanied by paroxysmal cough, a sensation of larynx spasm, cardiac arrhythmia and syncope due to hypotension

TREATMENT
Acupoints and techniques

Combination of points	Needles used	Insertion technique	Needling sensation
Hegu (LI-4, bilateral)	Two no. 30 filiform needles, 2 cun in length	Insert towards Houxi (SI-3) for 1.0-1.5 cun	Distending pain in the palm

Neiguan (PC-6, bilateral)	Two no. 30 filiform needles, 1.5 cun in length	Insert perpendicularly towards Waiguan (SJ-5) for 1.0-1.3 cun, taking care to avoid damage to the median nerve	Local distending pain and/or pain radiating to the dorsum of the hand and middle finger
Renying (ST-9, bilateral)	Two no. 30 filiform needles, 1.5 cun in length	Insert towards the spinal column to a depth of 0.5-1.0 cun; care should be taken to avoid the common carotid artery	Local distending pain or distending pain in the neck and throat
Lianquan (RN 23)	No. 30 filiform needle, 1.5 cun in length	Insert towards the root of the tongue for about 1.2 cun	Distending and heavy sensation in the root of the tongue

Method
- The patient adopts a sitting position, with the head tilted backwards.
- The acupoints are needled, with the needles being retained for 40 minutes; during this period, one session of needle rotation is carried out.
- Acupuncture should be performed once a day for ten consecutive days (one course of treatment).
- Recommence the therapy after an interval of five days if it is effective; otherwise terminate the treatment.

Clinical notes
Acupuncture is an effective therapy for treating glossopharyngeal neuralgia. In obstinate, frequently-recurring cases where acupuncture is ineffective, corticosteroid injection can be used. Provided that the insertion point is accurately localized and puncturing and technique are correct, satisfactory therapeutic results can generally be obtained by injection.

14 ACCESSORY NERVE PARALYSIS

The principal cause of accessory nerve paralysis is nasopharyngeal carcinoma. However, paralysis may also be precipitated by compression, involvement or irritation in or near the pharynx from such causes as diphtheria, acute and chronic pharyngeal infections, tumours, vascular diseases, syringomyelia, or lesions around the medulla oblongata.

Clinical manifestations
- simple accessory nerve paralysis is rarely seen
- in unilateral accessory nerve paralysis, the sternocleidomastoid muscle may weaken and atrophy; the patient is unable to move the chin towards the healthy side, but has no problems in movement towards the affected side
- in cases with paralysis of both sternocleidomastoid muscles, the head presents in forward flexion; in such cases, paralysis of the trapezius muscle is not significant, because its lower region is supplied by the 3rd and 4th cervical nerves
- in simple accessory nerve paralysis, only the upper part of the trapezius muscle is paralysed, which manifests as displacement of the shoulder towards the inferior and lateral sides
- when both upper extremities droop, the medial border of the scapula abducts with upper angle abduction being more significant than lower angle abduction

TREATMENT
Acupoints and techniques

Combination of points	Needles used	Insertion technique	Needling sensation
Tianyou (SJ-16, affected side)	No. 30 filiform needle, 2 cun in length	Insert towards the spinal column for about 1.5 cun	Local distending pain and/or pain radiating to the shoulder and back
Dazhu (BL-11, affected side)	No. 30 filiform needle, 1.5 cun in length	Insert towards the spinal column for about 1.2 cun	Local distending pain

Tianzhu (BL-10, affected side)	No. 30 filiform needle, 1 cun in length	Insert perpendicularly for 0.5-0.8 cun	Local distending pain
Hegu (LI-4, affected side)	No. 30 filiform needle, 2 cun in length	Insert towards Houxi (SI-3) for 1.0-1.5 cun	Distending pain in the palm

Method

- The patient adopts a sitting position.
- Unilateral or bilateral acupoints are selected according to the side or sides affected.
- The needles are retained for 40 minutes, during which time electro-acupuncture is applied to the acupoints on the neck, but not to LI-4.
- Acupuncture should be performed once a day for ten consecutive days (one course of treatment).
- Recommence the treatment after an interval of five days, if necessary.

Clinical notes

The therapeutic effects of electro-acupuncture are relatively good for treatment of simple accessory nerve paralysis to prevent atrophy of the sternocleido-mastoid and trapezius muscles and promote recovery of their functions. However, if there are primary diseases, they should be eliminated first before applying electro-acupuncture; satisfactory therapeutic results may also be obtained in this instance.

15 VAGUS NERVE PARALYSIS

Paralysis of the vagus nerve is characterized by functional disturbance or impairment of the vocal cords, digestive system and heart; this may occur due to a variety of factors.

The pathogenesis of the condition can be divided into two types:
- intracranial diseases such as meningeal tumours, chondroma, neurofibroma, metastatic tumours or flat cranial base;
- extracranial diseases such as cervical injury, parotid gland tumour and inflammation, sublingual gland tumour and inflammation, carotid phlebitis, carotid aneurysm and otitis media.

Clinical manifestations
- in unilateral vagus nerve paralysis, vocal cord paralysis and prolapse of the soft palate may occur on the affected side, accompanied by hoarseness of voice
- the posterior pharyngeal wall may be displaced towards the healthy side when the mouth is open because of paralysis of the superior constrictor muscle
- since the bilateral pharyngeal muscular fibres are interwoven at the midline, swallowing difficulty is not marked in cases with unilateral vagus nerve damage, but cardiac arrhythmia and tachycardia are often accompanying symptoms

TREATMENT
Acupoints and techniques

Combination of points	Needles used	Insertion technique	Needling sensation
Yamen (DU-15)	No. 30 filiform needle, 1 cun in length	Insert towards the infravertebral space of the 2nd cervical vertebra to a depth of 0.5-0.8 cun	Distending pain in the neck

Renying (ST-9, bilateral)	Two no. 30 filiform needles, 1.5 cun in length	Insert towards the spinal column to a depth of 0.5-1.0 cun; care should be taken to avoid the common carotid artery	Local distending pain or distending pain in the neck and throat
Lianquan (RN-23)	No. 30 filiform needle, 1.5 cun in length	Insert towards the root of the tongue for about 1.2 cun	Distending and heavy sensation in the root of the tongue
Neiguan (PC-6, bilateral)	Two no. 30 filiform needles, 1.5 cun in length	Insert perpendicularly towards Waiguan (SJ-5) for 1.0-1.3 cun, taking care to avoid damage to the median nerve	Local distending pain and/or pain radiating to the dorsum of the hand and middle finger

Method
- The patient adopts a sitting position, with the head tilted backwards.
- The acupoints are needled, with the needles being retained for 40 minutes; during this period, electro-acupuncture is applied to the points on the neck.
- Acupuncture should be performed once a day for seven consecutive days (one course of treatment).
- Recommence the treatment after an interval of three days, if necessary.

Clinical notes
Although involvement is extensive and symptoms diverse, acupuncture is effective in vagus nerve paralysis. However, if the disease is accompanied by lesions in the cranium or surroundings, the primary lesion should be eliminated before acupuncture is performed. The therapeutic effects are generally relatively good for simple vagus nerve paralysis with the function of the cervical muscle and cardiac rhythm being restored to normality reasonably rapidly.

16 HYPOGLOSSAL PARALYSIS

Paralysis of the hypoglossal nerve is characterized by declination and retraction of the tongue and dysarthria.

Paralysis is often caused by intracranial or extracranial diseases, such as cerebrovascular disease, cerebral tumour, or cranial or cerebral injury, and is generally one of the features of hemiplegia. Syringomyelia at the medulla oblongata, the early stage of amyotrophic lateral sclerosis, high-level cervical injury in the deeper region, tabes, or tumour or inflammation at the base of the tongue may directly or indirectly precipitate hypoglossal nerve paralysis.

Clinical manifestations
- unilateral hypoglossal nerve paralysis is seen more frequently than bilateral paralysis
- the tongue is extended towards the paralysed side and the affected lingual muscle is atrophic
- if the lesion is located in the hypoglossal nucleus, muscular fibre tremor can be seen in the atrophic lingual muscle
- functional impairment is not significant in unilateral cases
- bilateral hypoglossal nerve paralysis manifests as complete paralysis of the lingual muscles and retraction of the tongue at the base of the oral cavity, resulting in dysarthria, difficulty in swallowing food and dyspnoea

TREATMENT
Acupoints and techniques

Combination of points	Needles used	Insertion technique	Needling sensation
Shanglianquan: Located at the midpoint between Lianquan (RN-23) and the inferior border of the mandible (see diagram, page 199)	No. 32 filiform needle, 1 cun in length	Insert obliquely (at an angle of 45°) for 0.5-0.8 cun towards the root of the tongue	Distending pain at the root of the tongue

Taiyang (EX-HN-5, bilateral)	Two no. 30 filiform needles, 2 cun in length	Insert horizontally posteriorly towards Shuaigu (GB-8) for 1.0-1.5 cun	Distending pain in the temporal region
Hegu (LI-4, bilateral)	Two no. 30 filiform needles, 2 cun in length	Insert towards Houxi (SI-3) for 1.0-1.5 cun	Distending pain in the palm

Method
- The patient adopts a sitting position, with the head tilted backwards.
- The acupoints are needled, with the needles being retained for 40 minutes; during this period, one session of needle rotation is carried out.
- Acupuncture should be performed once a day for ten consecutive days (one course of treatment).
- Recommence the treatment after an interval of five days, if necessary.

Clinical notes
The therapeutic effects of the above method in the treatment of simple unilateral hypoglossal paralysis are quite good. However, since the majority of cases are a component of hemiplegia resulting from cerebrovascular diseases or cranial and brain trauma, treatment is rather complicated (please refer to the treatment of cerebrovascular diseases in the relevant sections of Chapter 2). The acupoints above can be used in combination with those for treating cranial or brain lesions. Restoration is relatively slow. Lingual paralysis gradually eases with simultaneous gradual improvement of hemiplegia and speech. Acupuncture therefore has a certain therapeutic effect regardless of whether the case is simple or is precipitated by cranial or brain lesions.

17 SPHENOPALATINE NEURALGIA

Sphenopalatine neuralgia, also known as Sluder's syndrome, is a severe pain occurring following stimulation in the area distributed by the sphenopalatine nerve.

The pathogenesis of the disease is not clear, but it is possibly related to infections in the nasal sinus involving the ganglion.

Clinical manifestations
- often occurs in women aged 30-40
- onset frequently occurs at night
- in most cases, the pain is located unilaterally at the root of the nose and the medial canthus, disseminating towards the deeper region and presenting as severe, burning pain
- the condition is often accompanied by congestion, conjunctival oedema, photophobia, scintillating scotoma or nasal mucous membrane congestion, rhinorrhoea or nasal obstruction
- an attack can last for 10-30 minutes, although in particular cases it may continue for up to two hours; sometimes it attacks periodically, three or four times a day, at other times, once every other day or even once every one or two weeks
- examination: significant tender points at the root of the nose and near the orbit or mastoid process

TREATMENT
Acupoints and techniques

Combination of points	Needles used	Insertion technique	Needling sensation
Yingxiang (LI-20, bilateral)	Two no. 30 filiform needles, 1.5 cun in length	Insert horizontally into the subcutaneous tissue towards Jingming (BL-1) for about 1.3 cun	Local distending pain

Yifeng (SJ-17, bilateral)	Two no. 30 filiform needles, 1.5 cun in length	Insert from each side towards the apex of the nose for about 1.3 cun; care should be taken to avoid the carotid artery and vein	Distending pain in the mandibular region
Hegu (LI-4, bilateral)	Two no. 30 filiform needles, 2 cun in length	Insert towards Houxi (SI-3) for 1.0-1.5 cun	Distending pain in the palm

Method

· The patient adopts a sitting position
- The acupoints are needled, with the needles being retained for 40 minutes; during this period, one session of needle rotation is carried out.
- Acupuncture should be performed once a day for six consecutive days (one course of treatment).
- Recommence the treatment after an interval of three days, if necessary.

Clinical notes

This therapy is effective in treating sphenopalatine neuralgia. The pain can generally be alleviated after three to five sessions. However, it can recur as a result of emotional factors or infection of the nasopharyngeal region or nasal sinus. The therapy can then be repeated, and similar therapeutic effects obtained.

18 **VESTIBULAR NEURONITIS**

Vestibular neuronitis is a condition characterized by dizziness due to inflammation of the vestibular nerve.

In the majority of cases, there is viral infection of the respiratory or alimentary tract, with the result that most authorities consider the probable cause of the disease to be viral infection of the vestibular nerve.

Clinical manifestations
- generally occurs in adults aged 20-60, and only occasionally in children
- onset is acute, often after waking up
- the disorder presents as acute, severe vertigo with nausea and vomiting, aggravated by opening the eyes and movement; in consequence, the patient is afraid to open the eyes or move
- often accompanied by spontaneous rapid nystagmus
- often confused with inner ear dizziness; the key point for differentiation is that inner ear dizziness presents with significant tinnitus and unilateral hearing impairment

Examination
- vestibular provocative test is abnormal bilaterally
- caloric test is abnormal
- rotation test is abnormal
- at the initial stage in some cases, there may be leucocytosis

TREATMENT
Acupoints and techniques

Combination of points	Needles used	Insertion technique	Needling sensation
Taiyang (EX-HN-5, bilateral)	Two no. 30 filiform needles, 2 cun in length	Insert horizontally posteriorly towards GB-8 for 1.0-1.5 cun	Distending pain in the temporal region

Fengchi (GB-20, bilateral)	Two no. 30 filiform needles, 2 cun in length	Insert and push towards the spinal column for 1.0-1.3 cun; as the skin at this location is thick, insertion should be made quickly with the needle then being pushed slowly to the required depth (thus avoiding bending)	Distending pain in the neck and/or pain radiating towards the ipsilateral occiput
Shuaigu (GB-8, bilateral)	Two no. 30 filiform needles, 1.5 cun in length	Insert horizontally posteriorly for about 1.3 cun	Distending pain in the temporal region

Method

- The patient adopts a sitting position.
- The acupoints are needled, with the needles being retained for 40 minutes; during this period, one session of needle rotation is carried out.
- Acupuncture should be performed once a day for six consecutive days (one course of treatment).
- Recommence the treatment after an interval of three days, if necessary.

Clinical notes

The therapeutic effect of this treatment is relatively satisfactory. The symptoms will generally improve after five or six sessions. After the disease is cured, it may recur and can be treated again with this therapy, achieving a similar effect.

Chapter 2

Cerebral disorders

19 TRANSIENT ISCHAEMIC ATTACK

Transient ischaemic attack (TIA) is a common acute cerebrovascular syndrome characterized by temporary local functional disorder of the nervous system due to transient ischaemia in the carotid and/or vertebrobasilar artery systems.

Clinical manifestations
- clinical manifestations depend on the location of the ischaemic attack; ischaemia in the carotid artery system should be differentiated from ischaemia in the vertebrobasilar artery system
- the symptoms and signs of TIA due to ischaemia in the carotid artery system are mild contralateral hemiplegia, unilateral sensory impairment, aphasia, visual impairment, or hemianopia, which lasts for a period ranging from several minutes to several hours and is followed by recovery
- TIA due to ischaemia in the vertebrobasilar artery system is often seen in elderly persons. The symptoms are headache at the occiput and transient visual impairment or visual field changes accompanied by brain stem symptoms, such as diplopia, dizziness, problems with articulation, difficulty in swallowing, facial numbness, ataxia or crossed paralysis
- cataplexy (sudden debility of the extremities) may occur, although the patient's mind remains clear; if cataplexy occurs while turning the head, it may be the result of impaired cerebral blood supply due to compression of the blood vessel by cervical spondylosis
- the patient recovers completely within 24 hours

TREATMENT
Body acupuncture
Acupoints and techniques

Combination of points	Needles used	Insertion technique	Needling sensation
Hegu (LI-4, affected side)	No. 30 filiform needle, 2 cun in length	Insert towards Houxi (SI-3) for 1.0-1.5 cun	Distending pain in the palm

Quchi (LI-11, affected side)	No. 30 filiform needle, 2 cun in length	Insert horizontally and push 1.2-1.5 cun towards Shaohai (HT-3) in the subcutaneous plane	Local distending pain
Qiuxu (GB-40, affected side)	No. 28 filiform needle, 2 cun in length	Insert along the bony crevice for about 1.3 cun	Local distending and stinging pain
Zusanli (ST-36, affected side)	No. 30 filiform needle, 2 cun in length	Insert perpendicularly for 1.2-1.5 cun	Local distending pain and/or pain radiating to the dorsum of the foot
Fengchi (GB-20, affected side)	No. 30 filiform needle, 2 cun in length	Insert and push towards the spinal column for 1.0-1.3 cun; as the skin at this location is thick, insertion should be made quickly with the needle then being pushed slowly to the required depth (thus avoiding bending)	Distending pain in the neck and/or pain radiating towards the ipsilateral occiput

Method

- The patient adopts a sitting or lateral recumbent position.
- The forearm should be rested on a flat surface with the medial aspect parallel to the body so that LI-11 and HT-3 are in vertical alignment.
- The acupoints are needled, with the needles being retained for 40 minutes; during this period, two sessions of needle rotation are carried out.
- Acupuncture should be performed once a day for ten consecutive days (one course of treatment).
- Recommence the treatment after an interval of five days, if necessary.

Scalp acupuncture
Acupoints and techniques
Motor area (unaffected side)
Location: on the scalp at the projection of the precentral gyrus. The line of the motor area is defined as its longitudinal central axis connecting the upper and lower points. The upper point is 0.5 cm posterior to the midpoint of the line joining antero-posteriorly the midpoint between the eyebrows and the highest point of the occipital tuberosity. The lower point is the intersection of the temporal hairline with the eyebrow-occiput line, which starts from the lateral end of the upper eyebrow and ends at the highest point of the occipital tuberosity (see diagram, page 200).

Selection of points: The upper fifth of the line is indicated for the contralateral lower extremity, the next two-fifths for the contralateral upper extremity and the lower two-fifths for the contralateral facial area.

Insertion technique: Relay puncture is performed after accurate selection of the acupoints. The number of zones used depends on the regions affected, as indicated above. After routine disinfection of the area concerned, the appropriate numbers of no. 30 filiform needles, 1.5 cun in length, are inserted quickly (to minimize pain) one after another into the scalp at an angle of 30° to the skin (one for each zone, selected in accordance with the regions affected). The needles should then be pushed down to the subcutaneous tissue, under the galea aponeurotica and moved horizontally along the cranium for 0.5-1.3 cun.

Needling sensation: local distending and stinging pain.

Sensory area (unaffected side)
Location: on the scalp at the projection of the postcentral gyrus. The line of the sensory area is defined as its longitudinal central axis, which is parallel and 1.5 cm posterior to the line of the motor area. Its division, selection of acupoints and relay puncture are the same as for the motor area line (see diagram, page 201).

Method
- The patient adopts a sitting position.
- Within 24 hours of onset of the transient ischaemic attack, body acupuncture is used. If limb function improves after 24 hours and the limbs on the affected

side are only partially paralysed or remain weak, scalp acupuncture is used as early as possible to improve cerebral circulation on the affected side.

- The acupoints to be punctured are selected according to the patient's condition. For example, if the features are impairment of motor activity and sensation in the lower extremities, the upper fifth of the motor and sensory areas are selected.
- Immediately after the needles have been inserted into the appropriate acupoints in the area(s), the needle shaft is rotated rapidly for one minute (approximately 200 rotations/min).
- The needles are retained for one hour, during which time three further sessions of rapid needle rotation (approximately 200 rotations/minute) are carried out for one minute every 20 minutes.
- After withdrawing the needles, press the points with a sterilized cotton ball to avoid haemorrhage.
- Acupuncture should be performed once a day for ten consecutive days (one course of treatment).
- Recommence the therapy after an interval of five days, if necessary.

Clinical notes

Transient ischaemic attacks are self-limiting, with recovery within 24 hours. By definition, the diagnosis of TIA can sometimes only be made once full recovery has occurred within the 24 hour timeframe. Most patients with TIA do not need any treatment and will recover with no sequelae. However, numbness and muscular weakness of the lower extremities, speech impairment, reduced powers of concentration, and dizziness may persist in some patients (for example, those with micro-embolism). In such circumstances, acupuncture should be applied early to obtain a relatively good therapeutic effect, particularly when scalp acupuncture is performed. Generally speaking, all patients will recover if acupuncture therapy is performed at an early stage.

20 CEREBRAL THROMBOSIS

Cerebral thrombosis is an acute ischaemic cerebrovascular accident characterized by local cerebral functional impairment due to ischaemia and anoxia when
the vessels are obstructed by thrombus.

Clinical manifestations
- often occurs in patients over 50 with a history of arteriosclerosis
- more likely to affect men than women
- onset is frequently seen after rest or sleep; in individual cases, onset may be
  slow and develop gradually over one to two weeks
- about 40% of cases have a history of cerebral transient ischaemic attack

TREATMENT
Acupoints and techniques
Scalp acupuncture
Motor area (unaffected side) See section 19, page 60.
Sensory area (unaffected side) See section 19, page 60.
Speech area no. 2 (unaffected side) Location: this line begins from a point 2 cm
posterior and parallel to a line starting from the parietal tuberosity and
stretches inferiorly for 3 cm (see diagram, page 201).
Speech area no. 3 (unaffected side) Location: a horizontal line on the scalp
with its longitudinal axis starting from the midpoint of the auditory area
1.5 cm superior to the apex of the ear and extending posteriorly for 4 cm (see
diagram, page 201).
Vasomotor area (unaffected side) Location: this area is defined as the line of its
longitudinal axis, which is 3 cm anterior and parallel to that of the motor line.
The upper half is indicated for oedema of the contralateral lower extremity and
the lower half for oedema of the contralateral upper extremity (see diagram,
page 201).

Acupoints for the relevant treatment area are selected as follows:
- for hemiplegia or unilateral paraesthesia, the upper fifth and next two-fifths
  of the motor and sensory areas are indicated
- for motor aphasia (when the patient understands written and spoken words,
  knows what he or she wishes to say but cannot utter the word – also known
  as ataxic aphasia, Broca's aphasia or expressive aphasia) with paralysis of the
  tongue and salivation, the lower two-fifths of the motor area are added

- for sensory aphasia (characterized by lack of auditory and visual disturbance but an inability to understand written, spoken or tactile speech symbols – also known as impressive aphasia, receptive aphasia or Wernicke's aphasia), speech area no. 3 is added
- for nominal aphasia (defined by the defective use of names of objects, i.e. the loss of the power of naming persons or objects, or of recognizing and recalling their names – also known as amnestic aphasia or anomia), speech area no. 2 is added
- for swelling in unilateral extremities, the vasomotor area is added

Insertion technique: Relay puncture (see section 19 for a description of the technique involved) is performed with no. 30 filiform needles, 1.5 cun in length, at the points selected above after routine disinfection of the scalp.

Method

- The patient adopts a sitting position.
- Immediately after the needles have been inserted into the appropriate relay puncture acupoints in the area(s) concerned, the needle shaft is rotated rapidly for one minute (approximately 200 rotations/min).
- The needles are retained for one hour, during which time three further sessions of rapid needle rotation (approximately 200 rotations/minute) are carried out for one minute every 20 minutes.
- After withdrawing the needles, press the points with a sterilized cotton ball to avoid haemorrhage.
- Scalp acupuncture should be performed once a day for ten consecutive days (one course of treatment).
- Recommence the treatment after an interval of five days, if necessary.

Clinical notes

The effect of this treatment is best in thrombosis of the middle cerebral artery, rather less effective in thrombosis of the anterior or posterior communicating arteries, and significantly less effective in infarction of the thalamus or cerebellum. In large cerebral infarctions and coma, the therapy cannot be performed until recovery from coma; although the therapeutic effects cannot be obtained instantly, they do appear subsequently.

Scalp acupuncture should be performed as early as possible once a definite diagnosis has been made, preferably within five days of onset. The longer the course of the disease, the less effective the therapy will be. In cases with sequelae of more than three and a half months, it is necessary to spend a relatively long time performing acupuncture to obtain satisfactory effects. In cases with contracture of the muscle in the hemiplegic limbs, the treatment is more difficult. In short, scalp acupuncture is a relatively good therapy for the treatment of cerebral thrombosis, but it should be used early.

21 CEREBRAL EMBOLISM

Cerebral embolism is an ischaemic cerebrovascular disorder similar to cerebral thrombosis. The disease is caused by embolic obstruction in the cerebral arterial circulation.

Cerebral embolism is often seen in the internal carotid artery, at the bifurcation or narrow section of the middle cerebral artery, or, in about 20% of cases, in the vertebrobasilar artery system. As soon as embolism occurs, infarction of the brain tissue develops at the area supplied by the occluded artery. However, the symptoms vary depending on such factors as the extent of the lesion, the presence or absence of collateral circulation, and whether or not arteriosclerosis is present.

When collateral circulation is adequate, the symptoms and signs of the disease may be absent or only present to a mild degree. In cases where an artery is suddenly and completely obstructed by an embolus, collateral circulation cannot be established immediately, cerebrovascular spasm often occurs, cerebral ischaemia is extensive and the symptoms are relatively severe. However, whenever the cerebrovascular spasm is relieved, collateral circulation established and the embolus has been forced to the distal part of the involved artery or is dispersed or dissolved, the extent of cerebral ischaemia diminishes and the symptoms become less severe.

Clinical manifestations
- embolism resulting from myocardial infarction or arteriosclerotic cardiopathy is more frequently seen in elderly patients and may be associated with mild disturbance of consciousness
- in young and middle-aged patients, an acute onset is often caused by rheumatic carditis or subacute bacterial endocarditis
- coma may occur when embolism affects the main trunk of a large artery or in multiple emboli
- headache, focal epilepsy, hemiplegia and aphasia may occur at the onset of the disease
- focal symptoms are determined by the artery affected
- apart from the features of cerebral embolism per se, there may be certain accompanying symptoms or signs, depending on the underlying cause of the thromboembolism, such as chest pain, dyspnoea, haemoptysis, or ecchymosis on the skin or mucous membranes

TREATMENT
Acupoints and techniques
Scalp acupuncture
Motor area (unaffected side) See section 19, page 60.
Sensory area (unaffected side) See section 19, page 60.
Speech area no. 2 (unaffected side) See section 20, page 62.
Speech area no. 3 (unaffected side) See section 20, page 62.
Vasomotor area (unaffected side) See section 20, page 62.
Foot motor and sensory area (unaffected side) Location: this area is defined as the line beginning 1 cm posterior to the upper point of the sensory area and 1 cm lateral to the midline and stretching anteriorly and parallel to the midline for 3 cm (see diagram, page 202).

Selection of points: The principle of acupoint selection is the same as for cerebral thrombosis, primarily in accordance with the symptoms. For example, the upper fifth and next two-fifths of the motor and sensory areas are indicated for hemiplegia or unilateral paraesthesia; for motor aphasia, the lower two-fifths of the motor area are added; for sensory aphasia, speech area no. 3 is added; for nominal aphasia, speech area no. 2 is added; for swelling in unilateral extremities, the vasomotor area is added; and for urinary incontinence and urinary frequency, the foot motor and sensory area is added.

Insertion technique: Relay puncture (see section 19 for a description of the technique involved) is performed with no. 30 filiform needles, 1.5 cun in length, at the points selected above after routine disinfection of the scalp.

Method
- The patient adopts a sitting position.
- Immediately after the needles have been inserted into the appropriate relay puncture acupoints in the area(s) concerned, the needle shaft is rotated rapidly for one minute (approximately 200 rotations/min).
- The needles are retained for one hour, during which time three further sessions of rapid needle rotation (approximately 200 rotations/minute) are carried out for one minute every 20 minutes.
- After withdrawing the needles, press the points with a sterilized cotton ball to avoid haemorrhage.

- Scalp acupuncture should be performed once a day for ten consecutive days (one course of treatment).
- Recommence the treatment after an interval of five days, if necessary.

Clinical notes

Scalp acupuncture is as effective a therapy for cerebral embolism as it is for cerebral thrombosis, especially in cases at the early stage. A good therapeutic effect can also be obtained once the underlying myocardial infarction or other serious disease has been relieved. Patients with a weak constitution or pulmonary infection or diabetes mellitus should be given the therapy in a supine position, because they cannot tolerate sitting for long periods or may faint during acupuncture. If fainting does occur, the needles should be withdrawn immediately and emergency measures should be instituted (put the patient in the recovery position and administer oxygen). During the period of acupuncture treatment, carers should be asked to encourage patients to undertake appropriate physical exercises to promote blood circulation in the affected side and enhance early recovery.

22 **CEREBRAL ARTERIOSCLEROSIS**

Cerebral arteriosclerosis is caused by a decrease in the cerebral blood flow, extensive brain tissue changes and impairment of the neural functions due to cerebral vessel atherosclerosis, arteriosclerosis and arteriolar hyalinization.

Severe extensive cerebral arteriosclerosis often induces a focal or general decrease of blood flow in the brain, resulting in cerebral anoxia and leading to cerebral atrophy.

Clinical manifestations
- occurs gradually, usually after 50, but occasionally in young persons
- affects men more than women (in a ratio of 2:1)
- often accompanied by systemic arteriosclerosis, and usually co-exists with coronary and/or renal arteriosclerosis

Main syndromes include:

Cerebral arteriosclerotic neurasthenia syndrome
- the patient often complains of headache, dizziness, poor memory, lack of concentration, slow thought processes, diminished ability to work, fatigue and numbness in the extremities
- often misdiagnosed as neurasthenia or functional disturbance of the autonomic nervous system

Cerebral arteriosclerotic dementia
- disturbance of memory and personality changes
- the patient's recent memory is defective, while long-term memory often remains relatively good
- the patient gradually loses a sense of time, location and subject, suffers from absences and slow reactions, and becomes apathetic and indifferent to the external environment
- personality changes include selfishness, obstinacy, morbid anxiety, delusion, infantile behaviour, changing moods, and paramnesia (false recollection of events that have never happened, or partial amnesia for events that have occurred)

Pseudoparkinsonism and pseudobulbar palsy
- increased muscle tone of the extremities, slow movements, and absent facial expressions
- involuntary crying or laughing and difficulty in walking where the patient also has pseudobulbar palsy

Subcortical arteriosclerotic encephalopathy
- chronic progressive dementia, cortical blindness, convulsive attacks, dysphasia, apathy, and unstable gait and involuntary motion

TREATMENT
Acupoints and techniques

Combination of points	Needles used	Insertion technique	Needling sensation
Taiyang (EX-HN-5, bilateral)	Two no. 30 filiform needles, 2 cun in length	Insert horizontally posteriorly towards GB-8 for 1.0-1.5 cun	Distending pain in the temporal region
Baihui (DU-20)	No. 30 filiform needle, 1 cun in length	Insert slightly obliquely postero inferiorly (at an angle of 15°) towards Houding (DU-19) for about 0.5 cun	Local distending pain
Shuaigu (GB-8, bilateral)	Two no. 30 filiform needles, 1.5 cun in length	Insert horizontally posteriorly for about 1.3 cun	Distending pain in the temporal region
Fengchi (GB-20, bilateral)	Two no. 30 filiform needles, 2 cun in length	Insert and push towards the spinal column for 1.0-1.3 cun; as the skin at this location is thick, insertion should be made quickly with the needle then being pushed slowly to the required depth (thus avoiding bending)	Distending pain in the neck and/or pain radiating towards the ipsilateral occiput

Method
- The patient adopts a sitting position.
- The acupoints are needled, with the needles being retained for 40 minutes; during this period, one session of needle rotation is carried out.
- Acupuncture should be performed once a day for ten consecutive days (one course of treatment).
- Recommence the treatment after an interval of five days, if necessary.

Clinical notes
Acupuncture is a reasonably effective therapy for arteriosclerosis, and works particularly well for patients at the early stage of the condition. It is especially effective for recovery of memory impairment, headache, dizziness, impaired concentration, fatigue and numbness in the extremities. Recovery is slow in severe arteriosclerosis presenting with dementia, morbid anxiety, delusion, infantile behaviour, changing moods and paramnesia, but a certain therapeutic effect can still be achieved.

23 LACUNAR CEREBRAL INFARCTION

Two-thirds of cases of lacunar cerebral infarction are induced by persistent systemic hypertension, which results in fibrinoid necrosis of arteriolar and capillary walls, hyaline degeneration, arteriolar atherosclerosis and atheroma, and constriction and obstruction of small end arteries. The remaining cases are induced by cerebral arterial atherosclerosis, narrowing or obstruction of the carotid artery, vasculitis, leukaemia, polycythaemia vera, metastatic carcinoma, or abscesses. These disorders may induce ischaemia, thrombosis or embolism of the end arteries, resulting in small foci of cerebromalacia.

Clinical manifestations
- long history of systemic hypertension
- about 20% of patients have a history of cerebral transient ischaemic attack
- some patients are asymptomatic after onset

The disease has the following five types:

Simple motor impairment
- mild hemiplegia affecting the face, arm and leg
- patients occasionally complain of paraesthesia without objective sensory disturbance
- the focus is located in the course of the pyramidal tract in the contralateral corona radiata, internal capsule and pons

Simple sensory disturbance
- paraesthesia or hypoaesthesia affects the face, arm and/or leg in one half of the body
- hemiparaesthesia is typically distributed strictly on one side of the median axis
- the focus is located at the contralateral thalamus sensory nucleus (ventral nucleus)

Sensorimotor disturbance
- unilateral debility of the face, arm and/or leg accompanied by ipsilateral paraesthesia or hypoaesthesia
- the focus is located at the contralateral posterior crus of the internal capsule and ventral posterior lateral nucleus in the thalamus

Ataxic mild hemiplegia
- mild hemiplegia is more severe in the lower extremity accompanied by obvious ataxia in the ipsilateral extremity

- patients occasionally complain of paraesthesia or mild hypoaesthesia in the limb
- the focus is located at the contralateral basal part of the pons

Dysarthria and hand dyspraxia

- central facial and lingual paralysis accompanied by dysarthria and choking during swallowing
- the focus is located at the contralateral basal part of the pons or the genu of the internal capsule
- pseudobulbar palsy, pseudoparkinsonian syndrome and dementia may also be seen, but they are rare

TREATMENT
Acupoints and techniques
Scalp acupuncture
Motor area (unaffected side) See section 19, page 60.
Sensory area (unaffected side) See section 19, page 60.
Speech area no. 3 (unaffected side) See section 20, page 62.
Foot motor and sensory area (unaffected side) See section 21, page 66.
Balance area Location: a line 4 cm in length extending downwards parallel to the midline from a point 3.5 cm lateral to the external occipital protuberance (see diagram, page 202).

Selection of points: The acupoints are selected according to the clinical manifestations. For cases with motor impairment in the upper and lower extremities, dysarthria and paralysis of the tongue, points in the upper fifth, next two-fifths or lower two-fifths of the motor area are selected as appropriate. For cases with paralysis in both legs and ataxia, puncture the bilateral motor areas, the upper fifth of the sensory area, plus the bilateral foot motor and sensory areas, and the bilateral balance area.

Insertion technique: Relay puncture with no. 30 filiform needles, each 1.5 cun in length; insert the needles into the scalp, one after another, at an angle of 30° to the skin (see also section 19 for a description of the technique involved).

Method
- The patient adopts a sitting position.
- Immediately after the needles have been inserted into the appropriate relay puncture acupoints in the area(s) concerned, the needle shaft is rotated rapidly for one minute (approximately 200 rotations/min).

- The needles are retained for one hour, during which time three further sessions of rapid needle rotation (approximately 200 rotations/minute) are carried out for one minute every 20 minutes.
- After withdrawing the needles, press the points with a sterilized cotton ball to avoid haemorrhage.
- Acupuncture should be performed once a day for ten consecutive days (one course of treatment).
- Recommence the treatment after an interval of five days, if necessary.

Clinical notes

Generally, the prognosis for cases with this condition is good and recovery is likely to be relatively rapid. However, where the symptoms described above occur repeatedly, then acupuncture therapy should be applied. Careful selection and location of the acupoints will bring about satisfactory therapeutic effects in a relatively short time. For persistent cases, the therapy will take longer to be effective, but satisfactory results can also be obtained.

24 SYRINGOMYELIA

Syringomyelia is a chronic and progressive degenerative disease caused by the formation of cavities (syringes) in the central portion of the spinal cord. Where there is an extension of syrinx formation into the lower brain stem, the condition is known as syringobulbia.

Clinical manifestations
- the disease occurs more frequently in men than women
- symptoms may appear in childhood or adolescence; however in most cases, the onset is between 20 and 30. The progress of the disease is rather slow, with clinical features being determined by the location of the syringes and their size

The clinical features and treatment of the disease differ according to the location involved:

1. Syringomyelia in the cervical and thoracic portions of the spinal cord
- frequently occurs in the lower cervical and upper thoracic portions of the spinal cord
- onset is slow
- the initial symptom is dysaesthesia of the hands; pain then occurs in a semi-horseshoe-shaped distribution in one or both upper limbs, chest and back, with a loss of sense of temperature in a horseshoe-shaped distribution
- progressive debility and atrophy of the hand muscles; this may gradually spread to the whole area of the upper limbs and the shoulder girdle muscles
- Horner's syndrome may occur when the ciliospinal centre at the C8-T1 segment or the pathway of the sympathetic nerve is damaged
- when pyramidal and spinothalamic tracts and the posterior cord are damaged by syrinx formation, corresponding motor and sensory symptoms and dystrophic changes will occur in the arm
- since the sensory tract of the trigeminal nerve extends to the cervical portion of the spinal cord, a loss of pain and temperature sensation may occur at the periphery of the face

TREATMENT
Acupoints and techniques

Combination of points	Needles used	Insertion technique	Needling sensation
Jianzhen (SI-9, affected side)	No. 30 filiform needle, 2 cun in length	Insert perpendicularly towards the inferior part of the shoulder joint for 1.0-1.5 cun	Local distending pain
Yunmen (LU-2, affected side)	No. 30 filiform needle, 1.5 cun in length	Insert slightly obliquely (at an angle of 15°) towards SI-9 at the posterior aspect of the shoulder for 0.5-1.0 cun	Distending pain in the shoulder and/or pain radiating to the arm and hand
Jianyu (LI-15, affected side)	No. 30 filiform needle, 1.5 cun in length	Insert and push slightly obliquely (at an angle of 15°) towards LI-11 for about 1.0 cun	Distending pain in the deltoid muscle and/or pain disseminating upwards
Quchi (LI-11, affected side)	No. 30 filiform needle, 2 cun in length	Insert horizontally and push 1.2-1.5 cun towards Shaohai (HT-3) in the subcutaneous plane	Local distending pain
Waiguan (SJ-5, affected side)	No. 30 filiform needle, 1.5 cun in length	Insert perpendicularly towards Neiguan (PC-6) to a depth of about 1.2 cun, taking care to avoid damage to the median nerve	Local distending pain and/or pain radiating to the dorsum of the hand and the middle finger

Hegu (LI-4, affected side)	No. 30 filiform needle, 2 cun in length	Insert towards Houxi (SI-3) for 1.0-1.5 cun	Distending pain in the palm
Xiaguan (ST-7, affected side)	No. 30 filiform needle, 1.5 cun in length	Insert perpendicularly for 0.5-1.0 cun, taking care to avoid the facial nerve	Local distending pain
Dicang (ST-4, affected side)	No. 30 filiform needle, 2 cun in length	Insert horizontally to join Jiache (ST-6)	Local distending pain
Taiyang (EX-HN-5, affected side)	No. 30 filiform needle, 2 cun in length	Insert horizontally inferiorly towards ST-6 for 1.0-1.5 cun	Local distending pain

Method
- Unilateral acupoints are selected for unilateral pain and muscle atrophy in the upper limb.
- In cases with bilateral involvement, bilateral acupoints are selected.
- Where there is only sensory disturbance in the area of the face innervated by the trigeminal nerve, select unilateral or bilateral points on the face (ST-7, ST-4 and EX-HN-5) with the addition of ipsilateral LI-4.
- Where the face and upper limbs are simultaneously affected, all the points on the upper limbs and face listed above should be selected.
- The forearm should be rested on a flat surface with the medial aspect parallel to the body so that LI-11 and HT-3 are in vertical alignment.
- After the needles have been inserted, electro-acupuncture is performed on the points for 40 minutes.
- Acupuncture should be performed once a day for ten consecutive days (one course of treatment).
- Recommence the treatment after an interval of five days, if necessary.

2. Syringomyelia in the lumbosacral spinal cord

- rarely occurs in this region of the spinal cord
- loss of pain and temperature sensation in the lower extremities, feet, perineum and genital organs
- muscular atrophy of the lower limbs and feet, marked dystrophy of the gastrocnemius muscle, and painless crepitus

TREATMENT
Acupoints and techniques

Combination of points	Needles used	Insertion technique	Needling sensation
Jiaji 16th (EX-B-2, affected side)	No. 30 filiform needle, 1.5 cun in length	Insert 1.0 cun into the fissure of the transverse processes of the 4th lumbar vertebra until a feeling like an electric shock radiating to the lower extremity is elicited	A feeling like an electric shock radiating to the ipsilateral lower extremity and foot
Huantiao (GB-30, affected side)	No. 30 filiform needle, 4 cun in length	Insert towards the piriformis muscle in the greater sciatic foramen for 3.0-3.5 cun, taking care to avoid damage to the sciatic nerve	Numbness radiating to the lower extremity and sole, or to the perineum and anus
Yinmen (BL-37, affected side)	No. 30 filiform needle, 2.5 cun in length	Insert perpendicularly to a depth of about 2.0 cun, taking care to avoid damage to the sciatic nerve	Distending pain in the thigh and/or pain radiating to the lower extremity and foot

Weizhong (BL-40, affected side)	No. 30 filiform needle, 2 cun in length	Insert perpendicularly for 1.0-1.5 cun, taking care to avoid damage to the tibial nerve, the popliteal artery and vein, and the peroneal artery	Distending pain in the popliteal fossa and/or pain radiating to the foot
Chengshan (BL-57, affected side)	No. 30 filiform needle, 2 cun in length	Insert perpendicularly for 1.0-1.5 cun, taking care to avoid damage to the tibial nerve and popliteal vessels	Local distending pain
Kunlun (BL-60, affected side)	No. 30 filiform needle, 1.5 cun in length	Insert towards the medial malleolus for 0.5-1.0 cun	Distending pain in the heel and/or pain radiating to the dorsum of the foot

Method
- The patient lies in a prone position.
- The acupoints are needled, with electro-acupuncture being applied for 40 minutes.
- After the needles are withdrawn, cupping therapy is performed for one minute.
- Acupuncture should be performed once a day for ten consecutive days (one course of treatment).
- Recommence the treatment after an interval of five days, if necessary.

3. Syringobulbia
- in most instances, this disorder is the extension of cervical syringomyelia towards the brain stem, but it can also exist in isolation
- the syrinx cavity is slit-like and asymmetric; only unilateral cranial nuclei or transmission tracts are damaged
- unilateral paralysis of the vocal cords and soft palate occurs, with atrophy and fibrillation of the lingual muscles

TREATMENT
Acupoints and techniques

Combination of points	Needles used	Insertion technique	Needling sensation
Shanglianquan: Located at the mid-point between Lianquan (RN-23) and the inferior border of the mandible (see diagram, page 199)	No. 32 filiform needle, 1 cun in length	Insert obliquely (at an angle of 45°) for 0.5-0.8 cun towards the root of the tongue	Distending pain at the root of the tongue
Yamen (DU-15)	No. 30 filiform needle, 1 cun in length	Insert perpendicularly for 0.5-0.8 cun	Local distending pain
Hegu (LI-4, bilateral)	Two no. 30 filiform needles, 2 cun in length	Insert towards Houxi (SI-3) for 1.0-1.5 cun	Distending pain in the palm

Method
- The patient adopts a sitting position, with the head tilted backwards.
- The acupoints are needled, with electro-acupuncture being applied for 40 minutes.
- Acupuncture should be performed once a day for ten consecutive days (one course of treatment).
- Recommence the treatment after an interval of five days, if necessary.

Clinical notes
At present, there is no specific treatment for syringomyelia. Acupuncture can alleviate pain, help to stimulate restoration of the atrophied muscles, and go some way towards eliminating the motor and sensory disturbances. However, the therapy will take a relatively long time. In cases with functional impairment of the limbs and muscular atrophy, patients should be advised to undertake physical exercise during the period of the therapy to enhance their general constitution and promote earlier recovery.

25 **PARKINSON'S DISEASE**

Parkinson's disease is the most common type of extrapyramidal tract disorder. It is characterized by tremor, rigidity and hypomotility and is caused primarily by degeneration of the substantia nigra and its pathway to the corpus striatum.

Clinical manifestations
- often occurs in patients over 50 years old, with approximately equal sex distribution
- can be a side-effect of certain psychotropic drugs
- onset is slow and the condition deteriorates gradually

The main symptoms are:

Tremor
- often begins in one hand
- rhythmic contraction and relaxation of antagonistic muscles at 4-6 times/ second appear in the involved limb
- the tremor accelerates with emotional excitement, decelerates when the mind is relaxed, and stops during sleep
- as the disease progresses, the tremor may spread to the ipsilateral lower limb and the contralateral upper and lower limbs, as well as the mandible, tongue and head

Rigidity
- the limbs become stiff and cannot move freely
- rigidity of facial muscles results in a decrease in expressional movement and makes the face mask-like
- severe muscular rigidity causes pain in the limbs

Hypomotility
- all movement is reduced in speed and frequency
- the patient often sits immobile, cannot undertake fine movements such as untying a knot, and writes in a progressively smaller hand
- speech is slow and monotonous with a low voice
- walking is characterized by small, shuffling steps, sometimes advancing with increasing speed (festinating gait)
- symptoms of salivation, increased secretion of the sebaceous and sweat glands, depression or dementia in some patients

TREATMENT
Acupoints and techniques
Scalp acupuncture
Motor area (unaffected side or bilateral) See section 19, page 60.
Sensory area (unaffected side or bilateral) See section 19, page 60.
Chorea and tremor area (unaffected side or bilateral) Location: a line parallel and 1.5 cm anterior to the motor area line (see diagram, page 201).
Indication: chorea and Parkinson's disease.

Selection of points: The acupoints for the motor and sensory areas are selected in accordance with the clinical manifestations (see section 19). Two points are selected along the chorea and tremor line.

Insertion technique: Relay puncture in the motor and sensory areas is described in section 19. Relay puncture in the chorea and tremor area is performed by inserting, at an angle of 30° to the skin, two no. 30 filiform needles, 1.5 cun in length, into the scalp inferiorly along the line for about 1.3 cun.

Needling sensation: Local distending pain is felt.

Method
- The patient adopts a sitting position.
- Immediately after the needles have been inserted into the appropriate relay puncture acupoints in the area(s) concerned, the needle shaft is rotated rapidly for one minute (approximately 200 rotations/min).
- The needles are retained for one hour, during which time three further sessions of rapid needle rotation (approximately 200 rotations/minute) are carried out for one minute every 20 minutes.
- After withdrawing the needles, press the points with a sterilized cotton ball to avoid haemorrhage.
- Acupuncture should be performed once a day for ten consecutive days (one course of treatment).
- Recommence the treatment after an interval of five days, if necessary.

Clinical notes
Parkinson's disease is a common condition. If the above methods are used at the initial stage, the therapeutic effects can be relatively satisfactory and the tremor can be alleviated or controlled without any drug treatment. In cases

where the disease has persisted for at least two years and the tremor appears either unilaterally in the upper and lower limbs and the head, or in all limbs, neck and head, the above therapy can only alleviate the tremors temporarily during the course of acupuncture treatment.

26 SYDENHAM'S CHOREA (CHOREA MINOR)

This condition is closely related to rheumatic fever. Most cases have a history of β-haemolytic streptococcus A infection one to six months beforehand or other manifestations of rheumatic fever such as arthralgia, erythema marginatum, purpura, or frequent sore throat; some patients may have rheumatic carditis before or after the onset, or in the course of the disease. Many cases have a family history of rheumatic fever. Spontaneous remission can occur two to six weeks after onset, but the disease may recur easily. Emotional factors and pregnancy may also contribute to recurrences.

Clinical manifestations
- often seen in children aged 5-15, more common in girls
- onset is generally slow, but may also occur abruptly with emotional stress
- at the early stage, the child is quieter than usual, cannot concentrate, exhibits emotional fragility, has clumsy movement, writes poorly and is liable to drop objects from the hand
- mild involuntary movements gradually occur in the face and fingers, such as frowning, winking, protruding the tongue, laughing, shrugging shoulders and extending arms
- involuntary movements can be aggravated by emotional stress; they disappear during sleep

TREATMENT
Acupoints and techniques
Scalp acupuncture
Motor area (unaffected side or bilateral) See section 19, page 60.
Sensory area (unaffected side or bilateral) See section 19, page 60.
Chorea and tremor area (unaffected side or bilateral) See section 25, page 81.

Other points

Combination of points	Needles used	Insertion technique	Needling sensation
Taiyang (EX-HN-5, bilateral)	Two no. 30 filiform needles, 2 cun in length	Insert horizontally posteriorly towards Shuaigu (GB-8) for 1.0-1.5 cun	Distending pain in the temporal region
Dicang (ST-4, bilateral)	Two no. 30 filiform needles, 2 cun in length	Insert horizontally to join Jiache (ST-6)	Local distending pain
Hegu (LI-4, bilateral)	Two no. 30 filiform needles, 2 cun in length	Insert towards Houxi (SI-3) for 1.0-1.5 cun	Distending pain in the palm
Quchi (LI-11, bilateral)	Two no. 30 filiform needles, 2 cun in length	Insert horizontally and push 1.2-1.5 cun towards Shaohai (HT-3) in the subcutaneous plane	Local distending pain
Zusanli (ST-36, bilateral)	Two no. 30 filiform needles, 2 cun in length	Insert perpendicularly for 1.2-1.5 cun	Local distending pain and/or pain radiating to the dorsum of the foot

Method
- The patient adopts a sitting or supine position.
- The forearm should be rested on a flat surface with the medial aspect parallel to the body so that LI-11 and HT-3 are in vertical alignment.
- If the symptoms are confined to the face and upper limb, select bilateral acupoints on the face and upper limb (a total of eight points).
- When symptoms appear in the face and all limbs, all scalp and body acupoints should be needled.

- For the scalp acupuncture points, the techniques described in section 25 should be used.
- For the body acupoints, the needles are retained for 40 minutes, during which one session of needle rotation is carried out.
- Acupuncture is performed once a day for ten consecutive days (one course of treatment).
- Recommence the treatment after an interval of five days, if necessary.

Clinical notes
The above depth of needle insertion is suitable for patients over 15 years of age. In younger children and thin persons, the depth should be shallower. Patients should be well prepared for acupuncture so that needling can be carried out in a co-operative atmosphere. Movements should be light and quick. The therapeutic effects are relatively satisfactory, and this treatment is especially effective and rapid at the early stage in cases with facial chorea only. In severe cases with chorea of the face and limbs, satisfactory results can also be obtained if the acupuncture is correctly administered and both doctor and patient are prepared to wait for results.

27 EPILEPSY

Epilepsy is a chronic disease characterized by recurrent paroxysmal disturbances of brain function due to neuronal discharges.

Various classifications of epilepsy are in use, but no classification is univer-
sally accepted. In this section, epilepsy is classified according to the clinical
manifestations of the seizures. Epilepsy can be a primary neurological disorder
(also known as functional, cryptogenic or idiopathic epilepsy) or may be secondary to an underlying brain disorder.

Clinical manifestations
Grand mal epilepsy (generalized tonic-clonic epilepsy)
- sudden loss of consciousness and generalized convulsion
  Aura
- malaise in the abdomen, dizziness, emotional instability or paraesthesia
  Tonic stage
- sudden unconsciousness, systemic muscular tonic contraction, head flexed
  posteriorly, bilateral flexed upper limbs and loud cry, dilatation of pupils,
  elevated blood pressure, temporary interruption to breathing, and cyanosis
  of the lips and skin
- this stage may persist for more than ten seconds before developing into the
  clonic stage
  Clonic stage
- rhythmic convulsion of all muscles, rapid at first and gradually slowing until
  the convulsion stops
- this period lasts for about one to three minutes
  Postictal stage
- respiration recovers first, followed by restoration of normal heart rate, reduction in blood pressure and a return to normal pupil size
- some 10-30 minutes may pass before the patient regains consciousness
- the patient does not remember the episode, and the aching and limpness of
  the limbs disappears within about three days

Minor epilepsy
- brief impairment or loss of consciousness. It occurs most frequently in children, and rarely in patients over 15 years old. The following subtypes are
  recognized:

Absence epilepsy
- sudden onset and termination of impaired cerebral function, a momentary break in the stream of thought and activities, which lasts for a few seconds, and may occur more than a hundred times a day
- during the seizure, the eyes are fixed or rotated upwards, the colour may drain from the face, activities and speech are interrupted, and the patient does not react to commands
- falling down is rare; after recovery, the patient does not remember the seizure

Myoclonic epilepsy
- attacks of intermittent clonus of bilateral muscle groups (lasting one or two seconds), especially those of the face and flexor muscles of the upper limbs, neck and trunk
- often complicated by grand mal epilepsy, less so by absence epilepsy

Atypical minor attacks
- most cases have diffuse brain pathology, and more than half of patients have mental impairment
- often occurs in children aged 1-3; similar to absence epilepsy
- duration is comparatively short, impairment of consciousness relatively mild, and onset of and recovery from the disease is slow

Focal epilepsy
- lasts from several seconds to more than a minute
- if it does not spread or progress into grand mal epilepsy, no obvious impairment will occur in mental activities

Two subtypes are recognized:

Motor attack
- clonic attack, characterized by a seizure initially involving one part of the body (e.g. mouth angle, eyelids, fingers or toes), progressively spreading to other parts of the body on the same side (Jacksonian epilepsy)
- aphasic attack or paroxysmal expressive aphasia
- rotational attack: the head and eyes, and sometimes the body, turn towards one side, or rotate in one direction. This type of epilepsy is liable to develop into grand mal epilepsy

Sensory attack
- body sensory attack: the seizures are predominantly one-sided and localized at one side of the mouth, tongue, face and extremities, resulting in paroxysmal numbness and stabbing pain
- special sensory attack, marked by hallucinations

Psychomotor attack
- may occur at any age, but later than other types
- disturbance of consciousness: in some cases, only paroxysmal, but in most cases other symptoms appear sequentially
- psychic symptoms: hallucinations and illusions, such as a feeling of 'gas rising in the stomach', déjà vu, loss of reality, and unreasonable fear
- automatism, marked by stereotyped movements, such as sucking, chewing, clearing the throat, rubbing hands, taking off clothes, or talking to oneself

TREATMENT
Group I: Emergency acupoints
Acupoints and techniques

Combination of points	Needles used	Insertion technique	Needling sensation
Shuigou (DU-26)	No. 30 filiform needle, 1 cun in length	Insert slightly obliquely upwards (at an angle of 15°) for 0.3-0.5 cun	Local distending pain
Shixuan (EX-UE-11, bilateral)	Ten no. 30 filiform needles, 0.5 cun in length	Insert in each finger to a depth of 0.1-0.2 cun	Local stabbing pain

Method
- The patient lies in a supine position.
- After the needles are inserted, each point is strongly stimulated in turn by manipulating the needle shaft until the patient regains consciousness.
- This therapy is indicated for emergencies only, and should not be used in normal circumstances.

Group II: Prevention of attacks
Acupoints and techniques
The following acupoints are selected for prevention of attacks and are indicated for cases with frequent attacks (for example, once to several times a day, once to several times a week, or before each menstrual cycle). Acupuncture is performed several hours or one week before the predicted seizure, or one week before menstruation, but only in cases where the time of attack can be predicted with precision.

Dazhui (DU-14)
One three-edged needle is inserted with a quick puncture into the centre of the acupoint for about 0.5 cun. Two other three-edged needles are inserted level with the point and 1 cm laterally on each side to produce bloodletting (by pressing the points with sterilized gauze in the other hand) after routine disinfection of the skin. After the blood has been cleaned, the points are covered with sterilized gauze held in place with a plaster for 10 hours. Avoid contact with water for 36 hours, if possible.

Shendao (DU-11)
One three-edged needle is inserted perpendicularly with a quick puncture for about 0.3 cun to produce bloodletting (by pressing the point with sterilized gauze). After the blood has been cleaned, the points are covered with sterilized gauze and held in place with a plaster for 10 hours. Avoid contact with water for 36 hours, if possible.

Changqiang (DU-1)
After the skin has been routinely disinfected and raised by the fingers, five three-edged needles are inserted to a depth of 6-9 mm in points 1.5 cm apart around the acupoint, with the pattern of the points taking the form of a plum blossom (see diagram, page 194). Press the point with sterilized gauze to cause bloodletting and treat as above.

Method
- The patient lies in a prone position with a pillow support under the lower abdomen.
- After the treatment, ask the patient to adopt a lateral recumbent position and rest for 10 minutes.
- The therapy is performed once a week for ten sessions (one course of treatment).
- Abandon the treatment if it does not work, or try it again after one month.

Group III: Convalescence
Acupoints and techniques
This group of points is used in the convalescent stage, or to consolidate the effect of acupuncture performed for patients included in Group II after the seizures have been brought under control. This group is also indicated for mild cases, such as minor epilepsy.

Combination of points	Needles used	Insertion technique	Needling sensation
Yifeng (SJ-17, bilateral)	Two no. 30 filiform needles, 1.5 cun in length	Insert perpendicularly for about 1.0 cun	Local distending pain
Neiguan (PC-6, bilateral)	Two no. 30 filiform needles, 1.5 cun in length	Insert perpendicularly towards Waiguan (SJ-5) for 1.0-1.3 cun, taking care to avoid damage to the median nerve	Local distending pain and/or pain radiating to the dorsum of the hand and middle finger
Jiuwei (RN-15)	No. 28 filiform needle, 1.5 cun in length	Insert inferiorly at an angle of 25° to the skin for about 1.0 cun, being particularly careful to avoid penetrating the peritoneal cavity in thin subjects	Local distending pain
Xingjian (LR-2, bilateral)	Two no. 30 filiform needles, 1.5 cun in length	Insert obliquely upwards (at an angle of 45°) towards the heel for 0.5-1.0 cun	Local distending pain

Method
- The patient lies in a supine position.
- The acupoints are needled, with the needles being retained for one hour without manipulation.
- Acupuncture is performed once a day for ten consecutive days (one course of treatment).
- Recommence the treatment after an interval of five days, if necessary.

Clinical notes
The causes of epilepsy are multiple and complicated. The three groups of acupoints indicated above for the treatment of the disease can achieve certain therapeutic effects. The results are relatively good for mild epilepsy and/or epilepsy with predictable onset. For treatment of cases with secondary epilepsy, the primary focus (primary and metastatic intracranial tumours, cerebral haemorrhage and mild craniocerebral injuries at the early stage) should be treated appropriately first. The therapy is only of limited assistance for patients with a long history of epilepsy, especially those taking anti-epileptics and tranquillizers and whose seizures are not well controlled. For patients taking long-term anti-epileptic therapy, the drugs should be gradually withdrawn during the therapeutic period as soon as the situation improves in order to avoid a rebound phenomenon and recurrence.

28 HYSTERIA

Clinically, hysteria is a common psychoneurotic or psychosomatic disorder resulting in temporary disorder of physical function.

Psychological trauma is the main cause of the disorder. The predisposing factors are determined in most instances by the patient's normal disposition, for instance unstable temperament, excessive mistrust, hallucination, inability to control the emotions, morbid self-consciousness and overweening self-confidence. If the above characteristics are not corrected in time, they will become predisposing factors.

Clinical manifestations
- clinical symptoms are extremely varied and present as symptoms of paroxysmal motor, sensory, autonomic or psychological impairment

Motor impairment
- motor functions of extremities are enhanced, weakened or lost
- pseudo-epilepsy, tremor, paralysis of the limbs (e.g. monoplegia, paraplegia, hemiplegia), curious gait (e.g. scissors-shaped gait)

Sensory impairment
- hyperaesthesia, hypoaesthesia or anaesthesia may appear over the skin in a glove or stocking distribution, not corresponding to patterns of sensory innervation
- characteristically there is an inconsistent pattern of neurological distribution, a sharp demarcation between the normal and involved areas, and, when the hyperaesthetic area is touched, the patient's expression is one of intolerable pain
- the patient may feel as if there is a balloon in the abdominal cavity that gradually rises to obstruct the stomach and throat, resulting in hiccups, a feeling of depression or asphyxia
- there may also be deafness, blindness (hysterical amaurosis) or aphonia
- a 'deaf' patient may be awakened from sleep by calling
- a patient is suddenly 'blind', but no ocular abnormality can be found on examination
- significant psychological symptoms before onset, for example, bilateral and symmetrical tunnel constriction of visual fields, or loud coughing from patients who are 'aphonic'

Autonomic nervous symptoms
- commonly presenting as vomiting, anorexia, urinary frequency, or pseudo-pregnancy

Psychological symptoms
- during an attack, such symptoms as laughing loudly and shouting, talking wildly and singing, dancing for joy, or exaggerated action or expression
- an attack is especially likely in a place where many people are present
- during emotional stress, some patients suddenly fall to the ground, fail to reply when addressed, and suffer systemic stiffness, trembling in all limbs and apnoea, similar to grand mal epilepsy
- an attack may persist for several minutes or hours

TREATMENT
Acupoints used during an attack
Acupoints and techniques

Combination of points	Needles used	Insertion technique	Needling sensation
Hegu (LI-4, bilateral)	Two no. 30 filiform needles, 2 cun in length	Insert towards Houxi (SI-3) for 1.0-1.5 cun	Distending pain in the palm
Zusanli (ST-36, bilateral)	Two no. 30 filiform needles, 2 cun in length	Insert perpendicularly for 1.2-1.5 cun	Local distending pain and/or pain radiating to the dorsum of the foot

Method
- Ask the patient to lie in a supine position.
- The whole process of acupuncture should be combined with psychotherapy; for example, keep the environment quiet, avoid mentioning hysteria, be understanding and friendly towards the patient, and persuade the patient to answer questions (age, the time discomfort begins, and so on). The possible underlying causes for the hysteria should be skilfully explored.
- Tell the patient in advance that acupuncture is about to begin. After the first puncture at LI-4 (the left side first for male patients, the right side first for

female patients), the patient should be able to speak; after the second puncture (the contralateral LI-4), the face should be relaxed and the eyes can open freely. After the third and fourth punctures (both ST-36), the whole body should be relaxed and the condition greatly improved.

- The patient should be told in advance that the needles must be retained for 20 minutes, even if there is a feeling of recovery, and that the therapy will require five further sessions to completely eradicate feelings of unhappiness, irritability and fear.
- Before removing the needle, the patient should be told that needle removal is painless and that there will be complete freedom of movement.
- The next five sessions of acupuncture are performed at the intervening period points (see below).

Acupoints used in the intervening period
Acupoints and techniques

Combination of points	Needles used	Insertion technique	Needling sensation
Taiyang (EX-HN-5, bilateral)	Two no. 30 filiform needles, 2 cun in length	Insert horizontally posteriorly towards Shuaigu (GB-8) for 1.0-1.5 cun	Distending pain in the temporal region
Neiguan (PC-6, bilateral)	Two no. 30 filiform needles, 1.5 cun in length	Insert perpendicularly towards Waiguan (SJ-5) for 1.0-1.3 cun, taking care to avoid damage to the median nerve	Local distending pain and/or pain radiating to the dorsum of the hand and middle finger
Jiuwei (RN-15)	No. 30 filiform needle, 1.5 cun in length	Insert inferiorly at an angle of 25° to the skin for about 1.0 cun, being particularly careful to avoid penetrating the peritoneal cavity in thin subjects	Local distending pain

Xingjian (LR-2, bilateral)	Two no. 30 filiform needles, 1.5 cun in length	Insert obliquely upwards (at an angle of 45°) towards the heel for 0.5-1.0 cun	Local distending pain

Method
- The patient lies in a supine position in a quiet room.
- The acupoints are needled, with the needles being retained for one hour, during which time the patient is asked to sleep; no needle manipulation is carried out.
- Gently wake up the patient before the needles are removed.
- Acupuncture is performed once a day for five consecutive days (one course of treatment).
- One course of treatment can be performed every month, if necessary.

Clinical notes
Acupuncture and suggestion therapy have an exceptional therapeutic effect in the treatment of this condition. The effectiveness of the therapy is determined by three factors: proper use of suggestion therapy, correct selection and localization of the acupoints, and quiet in the room in which acupuncture is performed. However, the most important factor is the success of the initial acupuncture, which is crucial for subsequent therapy to achieve satisfactory results; if the initial acupuncture does not work, there is very little chance of curing the patient. After recovery, the patient should be advised to do some physical exercises and keep a relaxed mind to consolidate the therapeutic effect.

29 MÉNIÈRE'S SYNDROME

Ménière's syndrome (endolymphatic hydrops) is characterized by paroxysmal vertigo, nausea, vomiting, tinnitus, progressive deafness, and a sensation of fullness in the ear.

The pathogenic mechanism is related to hydrops of the endolymphatic duct. Other factors may include fatigue, emotional stress or psychic trauma. The onset is between the ages of 20 and 50 in about three-quarters of cases, and men are affected more often than women.

Clinical manifestations
- recurrent attacks of vertigo lasting from minutes to days and attended by nausea and vomiting
- progressive sensorineural hearing loss
- tinnitus
- a sensation of distension of the ear

TREATMENT
Acupoints and techniques

Combination of points	Needles used	Insertion technique	Needling sensation
Taiyang (EX-HN-5, bilateral)	Two no. 30 filiform needles, 2 cun in length	Insert horizontally posteriorly towards GB-8 for 1.0-1.5 cun	Distending pain in the temporal region
Shuaigu (GB-8, bilateral)	Two no. 30 filiform needles, 1.5 cun in length	Insert horizontally posteriorly for about 1.3 cun	Distending pain in the temporal region

| Fengchi (GB-20, bilateral) | Two no. 30 filiform needles, 2 cun in length | Insert and push towards the spinal column for 1.0-1.3 cun; as the skin at this location is thick, insertion should be made quickly with the needle then being pushed slowly to the required depth (thus avoiding bending) | Distending pain in the neck and/or pain radiating towards the ipsilateral occiput |

Method
- The patient adopts a sitting position with the head supported.
- The acupoints are needled, with the needles being retained for 40 minutes; during this period, one session of needle rotation is carried out.
- Acupuncture should be performed once a day for six consecutive days (one course of treatment).
- Suspend the therapy if the disease is cured within six days.
- Proceed with the therapy after an interval of three days if it is working.
- Abandon the therapy if there is no progress after six sessions.

Clinical notes
The prognosis for this disorder is very good. Application of acupuncture can effectively alleviate vertigo at the acute stage. Vertigo can be improved or alleviated in many patients after just 10 minutes of acupuncture. Some patients are able to open their eyes, get up and walk after one treatment session. For cases at an advanced stage with multiple recurrent attacks, deafness and tinnitus, the therapy will take longer, but relatively good results can also be achieved.

30 ATHETOSIS

Athetosis is a syndrome characterized by myotonia and slow writhing, involuntary extension and flexion of the hands and sometimes feet.

Clinical manifestations
Athetosis
- affects limbs, either unilaterally or bilaterally
- at the early stage, athetosis is more manifest in the distal limb
- initially, there are constant, slow, sinuous and writhing movements of the fingers, the metacarpophalangeal joints are excessively extended and the fingers are twisted into a 'Buddha's hand' posture
- when the lower limbs are involved, the big toe is often spontaneously flexed dorsally
- when the facial muscles are involved, the patient often frowns and blinks
- when the throat and tongue muscles are involved, dysphasia, dysphagia and chewing difficulties may develop
- symptoms are aggravated during emotional stress, and absent when the patient is asleep

Increased muscle tone
- muscular tension increases while standing and decreases while resting
- in severe cases, spasticity can reach the degree of contracture, and when walking the patient may have a chicken-like gait
- symptoms disappear during sleep

Mental impairment
- the patient may present slow responses, clumsy hand and foot movements, and possibly dementia

TREATMENT
Acupoints and techniques

Combination of points	Needles used	Insertion technique	Needling sensation
Baihui (DU-20)	No. 30 filiform needle, 1 cun in length	Insert slightly obliquely postero-inferiorly (at an angle of 15°) towards Houding (DU-19) for about 0.5 cun	Local distending pain
Fengfu (DU-16)	No. 30 filiform needle, 1 cun in length	Insert perpendicu-larly to a depth of 0.5-0.8 cun towards the foramen magnum	Distending pain in the occipital region
Yifeng (SJ-17, bilateral)	Two no. 30 filiform needles, 1.5 cun in length	Insert perpendicu-larly for about 1.0 cun	Local distending pain
Hegu (LI-4, bilateral)	Two no. 30 filiform needles, 2 cun in length	Insert towards Houxi (SI-3) for 1.0-1.5 cun	Distending pain in the palm
Shenshu (BL-23, bilateral)	Two no. 30 filiform needles, 2 cun in length	Insert perpendicu-larly obliquely (at an angle of 75°) for 1.0-1.5 cun	Local distending pain
Zusanli (ST-36, bilateral)	Two no. 30 filiform needles, 2 cun in length	Insert perpendicu-larly for 1.2-1.5 cun	Local distending pain and/or pain radiating to the dorsum of the foot

Method
- The patient adopts a sitting position.
- The acupoints are needled, with the needles being retained for 40 minutes; during this period, one session of needle rotation is carried out.
- Acupuncture should be performed once a day for ten consecutive days (one course of treatment).
- Recommence the treatment after an interval of five days, if necessary.

Clinical notes
Acupuncture has a certain therapeutic effect in the treatment of this condition, although the duration of treatment is likely to be long. During treatment, the patient should be made to feel relaxed and happy. For cases with post-apoplexy athetosis accompanied by hemiplegia or bilateral paralysis of the limbs, scalp acupuncture can be used. In cases with progressive deterioration where acupuncture is ineffective, the therapy should be terminated and the patient transferred to a neurologist for treatment.

Chapter 3

Conditions of the spinal nerves

31 INJURY TO THE BRACHIAL PLEXUS

This disorder begins with symptoms of paralysis in the area of the brachial plexus distribution caused by external force or compression of the root or trunk of the plexus.

The main causes are fracture or dislocation of the shoulder, fracture of the clavicle, injury to the neck and shoulder during childbirth, cervical trauma, infection, sprain of the upper limb, or operations performed on the thoracic cavity. In addition, compression resulting from tumours or aneurysm may also cause paralytic symptoms of the brachial nerve plexus.

Clinical manifestations

Two types of injury to the brachial plexus are encountered, upper and lower. The upper brachial plexus type involves the 5th and 6th cervical roots (Erb's paralysis); the lower brachial plexus type involves the roots of the 7th cervical and 1st thoracic nerves.

Upper type
- motor impairment: the upper arm cannot abduct, the forearm cannot flex, the hand and arm cannot rotate externally, the forearm cannot supinate, and the hand is in line with the forearm – this is sometimes described as the 'porter's tip' attitude
- sensory impairment: although there is generally no sensory impairment, reduced pain sensation may be found at the acromion
- muscular atrophy: this may occur at the shoulder and upper arm or the muscles may be flaccid
- altered reflexes: hyporeflexia or areflexia of the biceps, triceps and radial reflexes

Lower type
- motor impairment: the fingers and wrist cannot flex, the fingers cannot abduct or adduct, the thumb cannot flex, adduct or abduct, or appose to the little finger at the palmar side
- sensory impairment: hypoaesthesia at the ulnar side of the forearm and hand
- muscular atrophy: the thenar and hypothenar muscles are atrophic
- autonomic nervous impairment: swelling and cyanosis of the hand, the fingernails become thin and fragile, and development of Horner's syndrome

TREATMENT
Acupoints and techniques

Combination of points	Needles used	Insertion technique	Needling sensation
Brachial plexus nerve point (affected side): Located on the lower neck, in the depression at the interface between the splenius capitis muscle and the sternocleidomastoid muscle (see diagram, page 183)	No. 30 filiform needle, 1 cun in length	Insert posteriorly to a depth of 0.5 cun towards the medial aspect of the posterior spine of the scapula (near the spinal column) in the direction of the first rib. Great care must be taken not to penetrate too deeply, otherwise the apex of the pleura and lung may be breached, leading to pneumothorax	Numbness migrating to the arm and hand, or a sensation like an electric shock
Jianyu (LI-15, affected side)	No. 30 filiform needle, 2 cun in length	Insert slightly obliquely inferiorly (at an angle of 15° to the skin) towards the elbow for about 1.8 cun	Distending pain in the shoulder or pain radiating down to the upper elbow along the median line of the arm
Shouwuli (LI-13, affected side)	No. 30 filiform needle, 2 cun in length	Insert perpendicularly along the medial border of the humerus for 1.0-1.5 cun, taking care to avoid damage to the radial nerve	Local distending pain and/or sensation radiating to the radial side of the wrist

Quchi (LI-11, affected side)	No. 30 filiform needle, 2 cun in length	Insert perpendicularly for about 1.5 cun, taking care to avoid damage to the radial nerve	Local distending pain
Waiguan (SJ-5, affected side)	No. 30 filiform needle, 1.5 cun in length	Insert perpendicularly towards Neiguan (PC-6) to a depth of about 1.2 cun, taking care to avoid damage to the median nerve	Local distending pain and/or sensation radiating to the dorsum of the hand and the middle finger
Hegu (LI-4, affected side)	No. 30 filiform needle, 2 cun in length	Insert towards Houxi (SI-3) for 1.0-1.5 cun	Distending pain in the palm

Method
- The patient adopts a sitting position.
- The acupoints are needled, with the needles being retained for 40 minutes; during this period, electro-acupuncture is applied.
- Acupuncture should be performed once a day for ten consecutive days (one course of treatment).
- Recommence the treatment after an interval of five days, if necessary.

Clinical notes
Electro-acupuncture has an excellent therapeutic effect in treating paralysis after brachial plexus injuries, especially paralysis caused by absorption of haematoma in the area supplied by the brachial plexus at the neck. A relatively good therapeutic effect can also be obtained if the injuries are in the early stage when brachial plexus injury occurs after reducing a fractured clavicle or a scapular fracture, or resection of a tumour or angioma. However, a complete cure is very unlikely for babies with delivery trauma. The condition may not be discovered until the infant is 1 or 2 years old and the child will probably not accept acupuncture until the age of 4 or 5 years. Long-standing brachial plexus injury may induce neuromuscular malfunction and so, even after applying very accurate acupuncture for quite a long time, neuromuscular function can only be partially restored.

32 BRACHIAL PLEXUS NEUROPATHY

In most instances, compression of the nerve roots of the brachial plexus is caused by cervical spondylopathy, prolapse of the cervical intervertebral discs, cervical tuberculosis, tumour of the cervical cord or vertebrae, fracture of the scapula or clavicle, dislocation of the shoulder, or arachnoiditis. Brachial plexus neuropathy may also arise at the level of the nerve trunk, which may be compressed in thoracic outlet syndrome or by a cervical rib, tumour of the neck, enlarged axillary lymph node (e.g. lymphoma or metastatic carcinoma) or fracture of the clavicle. Brachial plexus neuropathy may also be due to focal infection or inflammation of nearby tissues resulting from infectious diseases.

Clinical manifestations
- often seen in adults of weak constitution, after influenza or the common cold and where the neck or arm is affected by cold during sleep
- onset may be acute or subacute
- pain begins at the neck, shoulder and upper part of the clavicle, spreads rapidly to the posterior part of the shoulder, then within a few days to the upper arm, forearm and hand
- intermittent pain at the initial stage, becoming persistent and involving the entire upper limb after a short period
- the patient cannot lie on the affected side
- significant tenderness appears along the brachial plexus nerve trunk (at the supraclavicular and infraclavicular fossae or the axilla)
- pain is elicited on traction of the brachial plexus by abduction or elevation of the upper limb
- power of the upper limb is reduced in the initial stage
- tendon reflexes remain active at the early stage only, becoming hyporeflexive or areflexive after a short period
- in severe cases, swelling of fingers develops and the skin becomes atrophic and smooth

TREATMENT
Acupoints and techniques

Combination of points	Needles used	Insertion technique	Needling sensation
Tianding (LI-17, affected side)	No. 30 filiform needle, 1 cun in length	Insert towards the spinal column for about 0.5 cun, taking care to avoid damage to the external jugular vein and supra-clavicular nerves	Local distending pain and/or pain radiating to the upper arm and hand
Jianyu (LI-15, affected side)	No. 30 filiform needle, 2 cun in length	Insert slightly obliquely inferiorly (at an angle of 15° to the skin) towards the elbow for about 1.8 cun	Distending pain in the shoulder or pain radiating down to the upper elbow along the median line of the arm
Yunmen (LU-2, affected side)	No. 30 filiform needle, 1.5 cun in length	Insert slightly obliquely (at an angle of 15°) towards Jianzhen (SI-9) at the posterior aspect of the shoulder for 0.5-1.0 cun	Distending pain in the shoulder and/or pain radiating to the arm and hand
Binao (LI-14, affected side)	No. 30 filiform needle, 2 cun in length	Insert along the medial border of the humerus for about 1.5 cun	Sensation radiating to the radial side above the elbow
Quchi (LI-11, affected side)	No. 30 filiform needle, 2 cun in length	Insert horizontally and push 1.2-1.5 cun towards Shaohai (HT-3) in the sub-cutaneous plane	Local distending pain

Neiguan (PC-6, affected side)	No. 30 filiform needle, 1.5 cun in length	Insert perpendicularly towards Waiguan (SJ-5) for 1.0-1.3 cun, taking care to avoid damage to the median nerve	Local distending pain and/or pain radiating to the dorsum of the hand and middle finger
Hegu (LI-4, affected side)	No. 30 filiform needle, 2 cun in length	Insert towards Houxi (SI-3) for 1.0-1.5 cun	Distending pain in the palm

Method

- The patient adopts a sitting position.
- The forearm should be rested on a flat surface with the medial aspect parallel to the body so that LI-11 and HT-3 are in vertical alignment.
- The acupoints are needled, with the needles being retained for 40 minutes; during this period, one session of needle rotation is carried out.
- After the needles are removed, cupping therapy is performed for one minute.
- Acupuncture should be performed once a day for six consecutive days (one course of treatment).
- Recommence the treatment after an interval of three days, if necessary.

Clinical notes

Severe pain at onset is a typical symptom. This therapy is effective for most patients even where precipitating factors are relatively complicated. In severe cases, such as neuropathy caused by prolapse of the cervical intervertebral disc, the effect is satisfactory at the initial stage, but it takes a long time to eliminate numbness in the hand and upper arm. For severe prolapse, traction or massage therapies should be combined with acupuncture treatment. If there are other complications, such as pulmonary or cardiac diseases, they should be treated accordingly, and a good therapeutic effect can also be achieved.

33 **LONG THORACIC NERVE PARALYSIS**

This condition is characterized by muscular paralysis in the area innervated by the long thoracic nerve. Since the nerve is superficial in its course and is confined by the scapula and the anterior scalene muscle, it is liable to compression or injury, for example in thoracic surgery. Inflammation or tumour of the scapula or anterior scalene muscle can also compress the nerve and lead to paralysis.

Clinical manifestations
- slight backward displacement of the shoulder, including the acromion
- winging of the lower part of the scapula
- the scapula is rotated medially under the action of the rhomboid muscle and the levator of the scapula; its lower angle is separated from the thoracic wall, and the shoulder and scapula are higher than on the healthy side
- when the patient elevates the upper arm, the scapula lies close to the vertebral column with the angle of the scapula separated from the thoracic wall
- the angle of the scapula rotates anteriorly and laterally close to the chest

TREATMENT
Acupoints and techniques

Combination of points	Needles used	Insertion technique	Needling sensation
Xinshe (affected side): Located 1.5 cun lateral to the 3rd and 4th cervical vertebrae (see diagram, page 195)	No. 30 filiform needle, 1.5 cun in length	Insert towards the spinal column for about 1.0 cun	Local distending pain and/or sensation radiating to the shoulder
Renying (ST-9, affected side)	No. 30 filiform needle, 1.5 cun in length	Insert towards the spinal column to a depth of 0.5-1.0 cun; care should be taken to avoid the common carotid artery	Local distending pain or distending pain in the neck and throat

Jianjing (GB-21, affected side)	No. 30 filiform needle, 1 cun in length	Insert for about 0.5 cun towards the lowest third of the spine of the scapula	Local distending pain
Yunmen (LU-2, affected side)	No. 30 filiform needle, 1.5 cun in length	Insert slightly obliquely (at an angle of 15°) towards Jianzhen (SI-9) at the posterior aspect of the shoulder for 0.5-1.0 cun	Distending pain in the shoulder and/ or pain radiating to the arm and hand

Method

- The patient adopts a sitting position.
- The acupoints are needled, with the needles being retained for 40 minutes; during this period, electro-acupuncture is applied.
- Acupuncture should be performed once a day for ten consecutive days (one course of treatment).
- Recommence the treatment after an interval of five days, if necessary.

Clinical notes

Acupuncture therapy is quite effective in the treatment of long thoracic nerve paralysis. If the nerve has not been divided during surgery, the therapeutic effect is relatively satisfactory. In cases where the nerve paralysis is due to compression, the primary lesion should be eradicated first; reasonably satisfactory effects can also be obtained in these instances.

34 AXILLARY NERVE PARALYSIS

Axillary nerve paralysis is a complex of motor and sensory paralysis in the area innervated by the axillary nerve where the nerve is injured or compressed.

The main causes of axillary nerve paralysis are compression by a dislocated shoulder joint, fracture of the humerus, haematoma, penetrating injury to the shoulder, and pyogenic arthritis of the shoulder.

Clinical manifestations
- the upper arm cannot abduct to the horizontal level, extend forward or rotate externally
- the shoulder joint loses tension, and there is obvious lowering of the acromion
- hypoaesthesia occurs at the skin over the deltoid region
- at the advanced stage, the deltoid muscle will be atrophied

TREATMENT
Acupoints and techniques

Combination of points	Needles used	Insertion technique	Needling sensation
Jugu (LI-16, affected side)	No. 30 filiform needle, 1.5 cun in length	Insert obliquely (at an angle of 45°) towards the central point of the shoulder joint for about 1.0 cun	Local distending pain
Jianyu (LI-15, affected side)	No. 30 filiform needle, 2 cun in length	Insert slightly obliquely inferiorly (at an angle of 15° to the skin) towards the elbow for about 1.8 cun	Distending pain in the shoulder or pain radiating down to the upper elbow along the median line of the arm

Jianzhen (SI-9, affected side)	No. 30 filiform needle, 2 cun in length	Insert perpendicularly towards the inferior part of the shoulder joint for 1.0-1.5 cun	Local distending pain
Binao (LI-14, affected side)	No. 30 filiform needle, 1.5 cun in length	Insert towards the axillary region for about 1.0 cun	Local distending pain

Method

- The patient adopts a sitting position.
- The acupoints are needled, with the needles being retained for 40 minutes; during this period, electro-acupuncture is applied.
- Cupping therapy is performed for one minute immediately after the needles are removed.
- Acupuncture should be performed once a day for ten consecutive days (one course of treatment).
- Recommence the treatment after an interval of five days, if necessary.

Clinical notes

Electro-acupuncture has a relatively good therapeutic effect in treating this condition and is particularly effective for recovery of the atrophic scalene and deltoid muscles. However, the treatment is likely to be prolonged for muscular atrophy combined with relaxation of the shoulder joint. During and after treatment, the patient should be advised to undertake shoulder and neck exercises to aid recovery of the atrophied muscles.

35 MEDIAN NERVE PARALYSIS

Paralysis of the median nerve occurs as a result of compression of the nerve.

Common causes include injury or compression associated with fracture, direct compression or damage to the nerve from dislocation of the lunate bone, surgical procedures, neurofibroma of the nerve, excessive exertion of the wrist, or carpal tunnel syndrome. Neuropathy from systemic metabolic disorders (such as diabetes mellitus) may also result in median nerve paralysis.

Clinical manifestations
The clinical manifestations depend on the level at which the nerve is damaged:
Motor impairment
- wasting of the thenar eminence
- thumb adduction and opposition are weak
- if the nerve lesion is in the forearm or around the elbow, there is also paralysis of the long flexors of the thumb, index and middle fingers; on attempting to make a fist, the thumb and index remain extended, resulting in a 'pointing' hand
- limited pronation of the forearm

Sensory impairment
- hypoaesthesia or anaesthesia of the thumb, index and middle fingers, and the radial aspect of the ring finger

Autonomic impairment
- pallid or flushed skin
- the skin sometimes becomes dry, hyperkeratotic or very atrophic, and the nails become fragile and lose their normal lustre

TREATMENT
Acupoints and techniques

Combination of points	Needles used	Insertion technique	Needling sensation
Tianquan (PC-2, affected side)	No. 30 filiform needle, 2 cun in length	Insert along the medial border of the humerus at an angle of 75° for 1.0-1.5 cun	Local distending pain and/or sensation radiating to the wrist and hand

Quchi (LI-11, affected side)	No. 30 filiform needle, 2 cun in length	Insert horizontally and push 1.2-1.5 cun towards Shaohai (HT-3) in the sub-cutaneous plane	Local distending pain
Neiguan (PC-6, affected side)	No. 30 filiform needle, 1.5 cun in length	Insert perpendicu-larly towards Waiguan (SJ-5) for 1.0-1.3 cun, taking care to avoid damage to the median nerve	Local distending pain and/or pain radiating to the dorsum of the hand and middle finger
Hegu (LI-4, affected side)	No. 30 filiform needle, 2 cun in length	Insert towards Houxi (SI-3) for 1.0-1.5 cun	Distending pain in the palm

Method
- The patient adopts a sitting position.
- The forearm should be rested on a flat surface with the medial aspect parallel to the body so that LI-11 and HT-3 are in vertical alignment.
- The acupoints are needled, with the needles being retained for 40 minutes; during this period, electro-acupuncture is applied.
- Acupuncture should be performed once a day for ten consecutive days (one course of treatment).
- Recommence the treatment after an interval of five days, if necessary.

Clinical notes
Electro-acupuncture is effective in treating median nerve paralysis and the therapeutic effect is quite satisfactory despite the relatively long treatment required (generally, about three courses of treatment). For temporary paralysis caused by inflammation or compression by haematoma, the therapeutic effect is more evident and needs only about ten sessions (i.e. one course of treatment). The therapy is also of help in recovering muscular use and nerve functions follow-ing surgical repair of a divided median nerve, but it cannot produce a complete cure. Electro-acupuncture can also be effective in restoring hand function when there is chronic muscular atrophy following surgery.

36 ULNAR NERVE PARALYSIS

Common causes of ulnar nerve paralysis are compression at the elbow, fracture of the distal humerus (for example, at the olecranon), dislocation of the elbow or shoulder joint, tumour or inflammation. Compression of the elbow canal (elbow canal syndrome) is the most common cause.

Clinical manifestations
- the main manifestations are radial deviation of the wrist and weakness of wrist flexion, adduction of the hand, and flexion of the fourth and fifth fingers, which remain in an abducted position. When the two fingers are separated from one another, they take on a claw-like appearance
- loss of thumb adduction makes pinching difficult
- gripping objects between the fingers is awkward because of the difficulty in abduction and adduction
- in long-term cases, the lumbrical, interosseous and hypothenar muscles become atrophic
- the contour of the dorsum of the atrophic hand takes on a typical claw shape in severe cases
- hypoaesthesia or anaesthesia of the little finger and the ulnar border of the ring finger is evident

TREATMENT
Acupoints and techniques

Combination of points	Needles used	Insertion technique	Needling sensation
Shaohai (HT-3, affected side)	No. 30 filiform needle, 2 cun in length	Insert towards Quchi (LI-11) for about 1.5 cun	Local distending pain and/or sensation radiating to the little finger
Shenmen (HT-7, affected side)	No. 32 filiform needle, 1 cun in length	Insert slightly obliquely (at an angle of 15° to the skin) under the wrist crease and the distal aspect of the ulna for 0.3-0.5 cun	Local distending pain

Baxie (EX-UE-9, the four points on the affected side)	Four no. 32 filiform needles, 1.5 cun in length	Insert at each point and push proxim- ally along the metacarpal bone towards the wrist for 0.5-1.0 cun	Local distending pain

Method

- The patient adopts a sitting position.
- The acupoints are needled, with the needles being retained for 40 minutes; during this period, electro-acupuncture is applied
- Acupuncture should be performed once a day for ten consecutive days (one course of treatment).
- Recommence the treatment after an interval of five days, if necessary.

Clinical notes

Ulnar nerve paralysis can be treated with electro-acupuncture to give a relatively satisfactory therapeutic effect in most cases. However, the response depends on the severity and duration of the condition. In cases with mild damage (compression or irritation) and short duration, a good therapeutic effect can be obtained in a short time. For instance, at the early stage, an effective result can be achieved in 15-30 sessions if there is only weakness of the fourth and fifth fingers or slight atrophy of the hypothenar and interosseous muscles.

This therapy is also promising for cases with severe damage (direct nerve injury) and long duration with muscular atrophy and functional impairment in the ulnar nerve territory, provided that it is kept up for 30-60 sessions. After treatment, the patient should be advised to avoid elbow compression and to do hand exercises to enhance recovery of hand function.

37 RADIAL NERVE PARALYSIS

Radial nerve paralysis is a common neurological condition. The main symptom is paralysis of the extensor muscle group in the forearm, resulting in inability to extend the wrist giving rise to a typical 'wrist-drop' sign.

   The common causes are fracture of the middle third of the humerus or fracture of the forearm, dislocation of the elbow, inflammation (including systemic viral or bacterial infection or local infection near the radial nerve), chronic compression of the upper arm (such as sleeping with the head on the arm, which may compress the radial nerve in the spiral groove of the humerus), simple, surgical or penetrating injuries to the upper limb, compression of the anterior scalene muscle by tumour or haematoma in the neck and the region of the first rib, alcoholic neuropathy, or lead intoxication.

Clinical manifestations
- typical manifestations include paralysis of the extensor muscles of the wrist and fingers, hypoaesthesia or anaesthesia of the hand, the dorsum of the thumb and the space between the 1st and 2nd metacarpals, and wrist-drop
- in high-level injury to the radial nerve trunk occurring above the upper part of the upper arm, the elbow cannot be extended, the elbow cannot flex when the forearm and hand are pronated, and there is wrist-drop
- triceps muscle function remains normal if the injury is in the middle third of the humerus
- the functions of the brachioradialis, supinator and wrist extensor muscles are maintained if the injury is at a lower level, i.e. at the lower end of the humerus or the upper third of the forearm
- if the injury is distal to the middle third of the forearm, functional loss will be confined to finger extension and no wrist-drop will appear
- if the injury is at the wrist, there is only sensory impairment with no motor impairment

TREATMENT
Acupoints and techniques

Combination of points	Needles used	Insertion technique	Needling sensation
Shouwuli (LI-13, affected side)	No. 30 filiform needle, 2 cun in length	Insert perpendicularly along the medial border of the humerus for 1.0-1.5 cun, taking care to avoid damage to the radial nerve	Local distending pain and/or sensation radiating to the radial side of the wrist
Quchi (LI-11, affected side)	No. 30 filiform needle, 2 cun in length	Insert horizontally and push 1.2-1.5 cun towards Shaohai (HT-3) in the subcutaneous plane	Local distending pain
Shousanli (LI-10, affected side)	No. 30 filiform needle, 2 cun in length	Insert perpendicularly to a depth of about 1.5 cun	Local distending pain
Hegu (LI-4, affected side)	No. 30 filiform needle, 2 cun in length	Insert towards Houxi (SI-3) for 1.0-1.5 cun	Distending pain in the palm

Method
- The patient adopts a sitting position.
- The forearm should be rested on a flat surface with the medial aspect parallel to the body so that LI-11 and HT-3 are in vertical alignment.
- The acupoints are needled, with the needles being retained for 40 minutes; during this period, electro-acupuncture is applied.
- Cupping therapy is performed for one minute immediately after the needles are removed.
- Acupuncture should be performed once a day for ten consecutive days (one course of treatment).
- Recommence the treatment after an interval of five days, if necessary.

Clinical notes

If there is no neurapraxia and the nerve is intact, acupuncture will produce relatively good therapeutic results. If the nerve is partially or completely divided, the therapy is still effective, but will take much longer. Generally, muscular atrophy is relieved first; the radial nerve can partially recover its functions after a relatively long course of treatment. Surgery should be undertaken if there is partial or complete division of the radial nerve; acupuncture therapy is ineffective otherwise. Acupuncture is also helpful in the post-operative, recuperative period.

38 THORACIC OUTLET SYNDROME

Thoracic outlet syndrome is a complex of symptoms induced by compression of the brachial plexus and subclavian artery at the thoracic outlet.

Clinical manifestations

- often seen in women aged 30-50
- onset is slow; the initial symptom is pain, varying in degree from mild to severe
- in mild cases, there is episodic scapular pain that may radiate to the medial side of the upper arm
- in severe cases, wrist-drop is accompanied by numbness and a drilling, stabbing or severe burning pain; during onset, the pain is located at the posterior aspect of the scapula, and then radiates to the neck and the medial side of the arm, forearm and palm
- weakness and atrophy of the hand in adduction, abduction and flexion of the fingers
- if the thoracic outlet syndrome includes compression of the brachial plexus, sensory impairment may occur in an appropriate distribution (see section 31)
- the advanced stage is characterized by atrophy of the interosseous muscles and muscles on the ulnar side, decrease or absence of the biceps, triceps and radial reflexes, reduced skin temperature, paroxysmal pallor or cyanosis of the hand, and sometimes oedema of the hand
- in some patients, the majority of the symptoms occur at night
- X-ray examination may show a cervical rib or a long transverse process of the 7th cervical vertebra
- angiography may reveal constriction of the artery, dilatation of the artery at its distal course in the vicinity of the thoracic outlet, and the development of collateral circulation

TREATMENT
Acupoints and techniques

Combination of points	Needles used	Insertion technique	Needling sensation
Yunmen (LU-2, affected side)	No. 30 filiform needle, 1.5 cun in length	Insert slightly obliquely (at an angle of 15°) towards SI-9 at the posterior aspect of the shoulder for 0.5-1.0 cun	Distending pain in the shoulder and/or pain radiating to the arm and hand
Jianzhen (SI-9, affected side)	No. 30 filiform needle, 2 cun in length	Insert perpendicularly towards the inferior part of the shoulder joint for 1.0-1.5 cun	Local distending pain
Jianyu (LI-15, affected side)	No. 30 filiform needle, 2 cun in length	Insert slightly obliquely inferiorly (at an angle of 15° to the skin) towards the elbow for about 1.8 cun	Distending pain in the shoulder or pain radiating down to the upper elbow along the median line of the arm
Jugu (LI-16, affected side)	No. 30 filiform needle, 1.5 cun in length	Insert obliquely (at an angle of 45°) towards the central part of the shoulder joint for about 1.0 cun	Local distending pain
Quchi (LI-11, affected side)	No. 30 filiform needle, 2 cun in length	Insert horizontally and push 1.2-1.5 cun towards Shaohai (HT-3) in the sub-cutaneous plane	Local distending pain

Method

- The patient adopts a sitting position.
- The forearm should be rested on a flat surface with the medial aspect parallel to the body so that LI-11 and HT-3 are in vertical alignment.
- The acupoints are needled, with the needles being retained for 40 minutes; during this period, one session of needle rotation is carried out.
- Cupping therapy is performed for one minute immediately after the needles are removed.
- Acupuncture should be performed once a day for six consecutive days (one course of treatment).
- Recommence the treatment after an interval of three days, if necessary.

Clinical notes

Acupuncture is very effective in treating thoracic outlet syndrome. Nocturnal pain can generally be lessened or alleviated after three to five sessions. However, for cases with severe compression, the therapy should be combined with resection of the cervical rib or the anterior scalene muscle. The remaining sequelae can also be treated by acupuncture; the therapeutic effect is relatively satisfactory. Electro-acupuncture is also effective for chronic cases of post-operative muscular atrophy.

39 SUPERIOR CLUNIAL NERVE INJURY

Superior clunial nerve injury is characterized by pain in the superior part of the buttock.

The main cause of this injury is excessive traction on the nerve due to sudden and forceful rotation of the trunk. This leads to inflammation, congestion and swelling during the acute stage, and to proliferation of tissues around the nerve and neurofibrillar degeneration during the chronic stage.

In the majority of cases, there is abnormality of the contour of the iliac crest; its excessive height or extroversion allows nerve damage to occur more easily. In cases with chronic damage, the superior clunial nerve increases in diameter and becomes cord-like.

Clinical manifestations
- often occurs in males aged 20-40
- generally unilateral
- the patient often has a history of strenuous exercise or sprain
- in cases with severe sprain, fierce pain will occur from the very beginning
- radiating, stabbing, distending or lacerating pain may occur at the region distributed by the nerve when the patient flexes or slightly rotates the waist, lies down, sits down or stands up
- the patient feels as though there is no strength at the waist when getting into bed, sitting down or standing up

Examination
- tenderness is marked at the highest point of the posterior iliac crest
- a cord-like structure is palpable at the gluteal region below the tender point; when the region is pressed, the pain at the gluteal and iliac crest region becomes aggravated

TREATMENT
Acupoints and techniques

Combination of points	Needles used	Insertion technique	Needling sensation
Yaoyi (EX-B-6, affected side)	Two no. 30 filiform needles, 1.5 cun in length	Insert the needles to a depth of 0.8-1.2 cun; the first needle is inserted obliquely (at an angle of 45°) towards the central part of the lower buttock, whereas the second one is inserted perpendicularly along the posterior superior iliac spine	The needling response for the first puncture radiates to the buttock, the posterior aspect of the thigh and the popliteal region; for the second needle, there is local distending pain in the lower back
Tunzhong (affected side): Taking a line between the greater trochanter and the ischial tuberosity as the base of an equilateral triangle, Tunzhong is located at the apex of the triangle (see diagram, page 196)	No. 30 filiform needle, 3 cun in length	Insert perpendicularly to a depth of about 2.0 cun	Local distending pain and/or sensation radiating to the lower extremity
Weizhong (BL-40, affected side)	No. 30 filiform needle, 2 cun in length	Insert perpendicularly for 1.0-1.5 cun, taking care to avoid damage to the tibial nerve, the popliteal artery and vein, and the peroneal artery	Distending pain in the popliteal fossa and/or pain radiating to the foot

Method

- The patient lies in a prone position.
- The acupoints are needled, with the needles being retained for 40 minutes; during this period, one session of needle rotation is carried out.
- After the needles are removed, cupping therapy is performed for one minute.
- Acupuncture should be performed once a day for six consecutive days (one course of treatment).
- Recommence the treatment after an interval of five days, if necessary.

Clinical notes

During the acute stage of the condition, treatment using the above methods has a good therapeutic effect; the pain can generally be relieved in about six sessions (i.e. one course of treatment). Satisfactory therapeutic effects can also be obtained in chronic cases, where there is significant prominence at the iliac crest and a relatively large, cord-like structure at the buttock. However, treatment of these cases requires a longer time, and corticosteroid injection at the tender point should be considered; care should be taken to avoid damaging the nerve by the injection.

40 SCIATICA

Sciatica refers to pain in the course of the sciatic nerve and its branches; it is a common peripheral nerve condition, usually seen in young men.

Clinical manifestations
- usually unilateral, presenting with an acute or subacute onset
- clinically, the disease is divided into three types – root, trunk and plexus – depending on the site of the lesion

Root
- commonly seen in patients with lumbar spondylosis, intervertebral disc lesion, or stenosis of the vertebral canal
- acute onset with significant sprain history in the majority of cases
- in the early stages, the pain is located at the lumbar and hip regions within the distribution of the sciatic nerve, gradually spreading to the posterior aspect of the thigh, the popliteal area and leg, and the lateral and plantar surfaces of the foot
- significant tender points in the lumbar region when the nerve root is stimulated (1 cun lateral to the 3rd-5th lumbar vertebrae)
- numbness of the lateral surface of the leg and the sole is present in severe cases

Trunk
- frequently seen in cases with inflammation at the exit of the nerve from the pelvic cavity
- gradual onset
- pain and tenderness in the piriformis area at the onset, gradually extending to the posterior aspect of the thigh, the popliteal region, and the lateral aspect of the lower leg and foot, but pain does not occur in the loin
- numbness of the sole may occur in severe cases

Plexus
- frequently seen in female patients with lesions in the pelvic cavity, such as pelvic inflammation, adnexitis or tumours
- clinically, the majority of cases exhibit significant symptoms in the lower abdominal cavity, accompanied by pain along the distribution of the sciatic nerve
- neuralgia of the superior gluteal, femoral and obturator nerves coexists in some cases

TREATMENT
Acupoints and techniques

Combination of points	Needles used	Insertion technique	Needling sensation
Qihaishu (BL-24, affected side)	No. 28 filiform needle, 2 cun in length	Insert perpendicularly for about 1.0-1.5 cun	Numbness and distending sensation radiating to the lower extremity and the sole
Zhibian (BL-54, affected side)	No. 28 filiform needle, 3 cun in length	Insert perpendicularly towards the greater sciatic foramen for about 2.8 cun	Distending pain and/or pain radiating to the lower extremity
Huantiao (GB-30, affected side)	No. 28 filiform needle, 4 cun in length	Insert towards the greater sciatic foramen for 3.0-3.5 cun, taking care to avoid damage to the sciatic nerve	Local distending pain or electric shock-like sensation radiating to the ipsilateral lower limb
Yinmen (BL-37, affected side)	No. 30 filiform needle, 2.5 cun in length	Insert perpendicularly to a depth of about 2.0 cun, taking care to avoid damage to the sciatic nerve	Distending pain in the thigh and/or pain radiating to the lower extremity and foot
Weizhong (BL-40, affected side)	No. 30 filiform needle, 1.5 cun in length	Insert slightly obliquely upwards (at an angle of 15°) for about 1.0 cun, taking care to avoid damage to the tibial nerve and popliteal vessels	Distending pain in the popliteal fossa

Chengshan (BL-57, affected side)	No. 30 filiform needle, 2 cun in length	Insert perpendicularly for 1.0-1.5 cun, taking care to avoid damage to the tibial nerve and popliteal vessels	Local distending pain
Kunlun (BL-60, affected side)	No. 30 filiform needle, 1.5 cun in length	Insert towards the medial malleolus for 0.5-1.0 cun	Distending pain in the heel and/or pain radiating to the dorsum of the foot

Method

- The patient lies in a prone position.
- The acupoints are needled, with the needles being rotained for 10 minutes, during this period, one session of needle rotation is carried out.
- Cupping therapy is performed for one minute immediately after the needles are removed.
- Acupuncture should be performed once a day for ten consecutive days (one course of treatment).
- Recommence the treatment after an interval of five days, if necessary.

Clinical notes

Acupuncture therapy produces satisfactory results in the treatment of sciatica, except for cases with serious prolapse of the intervertebral disc and lumbar spondylosis. In cases with secondary sciatica, the underlying cause should be relieved first before applying the above methods; results are also satisfactory in these instances. In cases with underlying infection, antibiotics should be used to treat the infection and reduce inflammation; if acupuncture treatment takes place at the same time, it is also possible to achieve reasonable therapeutic effects.

41 OBTURATOR NERVE INJURY

Obturator nerve injury is characterized by weak adduction of the thigh and limitation of foot abduction due to trauma, compression or irritation of the obturator nerve.

The causes of this injury include trauma to the nerve in the medial muscular group of the thigh, compression or irritation of the nerve by pelvic tumour, inflammation or femoral hernia, or surgical trauma.

Clinical manifestations
- adduction of the thigh is limited
- the foot is slightly abducted
- difficulty in placing the affected foot on the dorsum of the healthy one

TREATMENT
Acupoints and techniques

Combination of points	Needles used	Insertion technique	Needling sensation
Zuwuli (LR-10, affected side)	No. 30 filiform needle, 2 cun in length	Insert perpendicularly to a depth of about 1.5 cun, taking particular care to avoid damage to the femoral artery and vein	Local distending pain
Jimen (SP-11, affected side)	No. 30 filiform needle, 1.5 cun in length	Insert towards the femur for about 1.0 cun, taking care to avoid damage to the femoral artery and vein, and the saphenous nerve	Local distending pain and/or pain radiating to the medial side of the leg

Futu (ST-32, affected side)	No. 30 filiform needle, 2 cun in length	Insert towards the medial aspect of the femur for about 1.8 cun	Local distending pain
Xuehai (SP-10, affected side)	No. 30 filiform needle, 2 cun in length	Insert perpendicularly for about 1.5 cun	Local distending pain

Method

- The patient lies in a supine position.
- The acupoints are needled, with the needles being retained for 40 minutes; during this period, electro-acupuncture is applied.
- Cupping therapy is performed for one minute immediately after the needles are removed.
- Acupuncture should be performed once a day for ten consecutive days (one course of treatment).
- Recommence the treatment after an interval of five days, if necessary.

Clinical notes

The therapeutic effect of acupuncture treatment is good when the duration of compression is short, the obturator nerve injury is incomplete, and the primary cause has been relieved. If the obturator nerve is seriously damaged (for example, where there is severe compression of the nerve due to tumour of the pelvic cavity) with major impairment of nerve function, it will be necessary to continue the therapy for a relatively long period; however, a satisfactory result can also be obtained if acupuncture is performed accurately and meticulously.

42 TIBIAL NERVE INJURY

Injury to the tibial nerve can result from a number of causes, the most common being perforating injuries, compression by tumour or cyst in the popliteal fossa, and strenuous physical exercise (such as jumping and sprinting). In addition, diabetes mellitus, polyarteritis nodosa and idiopathic tibial neuritis may induce paralysis.

Clinical manifestations
- in complete tibial nerve paralysis (injury at the popliteal region), a 'claw-foot' appears
- dysaesthesia is present at the posterior aspect of the leg, the lateral border of the foot, the lateral part of the heel, and the medial and lateral part of the sole
- some patients may experience a burning pain
- where the tibial nerve is only partially injured, pain varying from mild to severe is located at the posterior aspect of the leg and radiates to the medial part of the metatarsus
- in severe cases, the pain can involve the entire lower extremity and is accompanied by vasomotor and sudomotor impairment, together with trophic changes

TREATMENT
Acupoints and techniques

Combination of points	Needles used	Insertion technique	Needling sensation
Weizhong (BL-40, affected side)	No. 30 filiform needle, 2 cun in length	Insert slightly obliquely upwards (at an angle of 15°) towards the medial border of the femur for 1.5 cun	Local distending pain and/or pain radiating to the leg and the sole
Chengshan (BL-57, affected side)	No. 30 filiform needle, 2 cun in length	Insert perpendicularly for 1.0-1.5 cun, taking care to avoid damage to the tibial nerve and popliteal vessels	Local distending pain

Sanyinjiao (SP-6, affected side)	No. 30 filiform needle, 2 cun in length	Insert towards Xuanzhong (GB-39) for 1.0-1.5 cun	Local distending pain
Bafeng (EX-LE-10, four points on the affected side)	Four no. 30 filiform needles, 1.5 cun in length	Insert obliquely upwards (at an angle of 45°) for 0.5-1.0 cun	Local distending pain

Method

- The patient adopts a sitting position.
- The acupoints are needled, with the needles being retained for 40 minutes.
- Acupuncture should be performed once a day for ten consecutive days (one course of treatment)
- Recommence the treatment after an interval of five days, if necessary.

Clinical notes

In cases with tibial nerve injury manifesting only as pain and numbness in the lower extremity, acupuncture has a relatively rapid therapeutic effect; both pain and numbness can generally be alleviated after about six sessions. If the injury and tibial nerve paralysis are of short duration and the nerve has not been separated, the therapeutic effect is also quite good and recovery will be rapid. Where the nerve has been divided for a relatively long time and the muscles are atrophic, it is necessary to persist with the therapy for longer; however, satisfactory results may also be obtained by careful and accurate treatment combined with massage of the soleus and gastrocnemius muscles and the sole, and active, forceful plantarflexion of the foot.

43 PARALYSIS OF THE COMMON PERONEAL NERVE

Direct and indirect injuries to the common peroneal nerve are caused by long-term compression, trauma or pressure at the head of the fibula, neuritis, traction, local infection complicating diabetes, and intoxication by alcohol or organophosphorus pesticides. Compression may be due to prolonged squatting, sitting cross-legged, or pressure from incorrectly applied bandages or casts on the lower leg.

Clinical manifestations
- typical foot-drop
- flexion of the dorsum of the foot, toes pointing upwards
- inability to abduct or invert the affected foot, talipes varus, talipes equinus
- in chronic cases, the condition will develop into talipes equinovarus, with a gait similar to that of a chicken
- the muscle group of the anterolateral aspect of the lower leg is atrophic, but the Achilles tendon reflex is unaffected
- the tibialis anterior muscle is paralysed, resulting in flexion of the dorsum of the foot, difficulty in elevating the medial border of the foot and slightly abducted foot-drop

TREATMENT
Acupoints and techniques

Combination of points	Needles used	Insertion technique	Needling sensation
Common peroneal nerve point (affected side): Located below the knee on the lateral border of the fibula and 0.5 cun inferior to the head of the fibula (see diagram, page 198)	No. 30 filiform needle, 2 cun in length	Insert perpendicularly for 1.0-1.5 cun	Local distending pain and/or pain radiating to the dorsum of the foot

Zusanli (ST-36, affected side)	No. 30 filiform needle, 2 cun in length	Insert perpendicularly for 1.2-1.5 cun	Local distending pain and/or pain radiating to the dorsum of the foot
Xingjian (LR-2, affected side)	No. 30 filiform needle, 1.5 cun in length	Insert obliquely upwards (at an angle of 45°) towards the heel for 0.5-1.0 cun	Local distending pain
Neiting (ST-44, affected side)	No. 30 filiform needle, 1.5 cun in length	Insert obliquely upwards (at an angle of 45°) for about 1.0 cun	Local distending pain

Method

- The patient adopts a sitting position.
- The acupoints are needled, with the needles being retained for 40 minutes; during this period, electro-acupuncture is applied.
- Acupuncture should be performed once a day for ten consecutive days (one course of treatment).
- Recommence the treatment after an interval of five days, if necessary.

Clinical notes

The therapeutic effect of acupuncture is relatively good if the injury is mild with a short history and there is no division of the nerve and no muscular atrophy. Where there has been prolonged compression and the muscles are atrophic, this therapy can produce a certain effect if it is performed for a long period. Surgical treatment should be undertaken where the nerve has been divided, because acupuncture can only partially restore muscular tension in some muscles. The patient's confidence in this therapy is also an important factor in its success. Massage of the tibialis anterior muscle and the dorsum and sole of the foot, stretching of the dorsum of the foot and correction of gait to the normal walking posture will enhance early recovery of the affected leg.

44 FEMORAL NERVE PARALYSIS

Femoral nerve paralysis is characterized by paralysis and malfunction of the muscles in the area innervated by the nerve.

The causes of femoral nerve paralysis are multiple and include tumours in the pelvis, spinal cord, vertebral column and retroperitoneum, surgical trauma and injury in the inguinal region and pelvis, abscess or haematoma of the psoas major muscle, aneurysm of the femoral artery, diabetic neuropathy, lead intoxication, and improper posture of the body, such as excessive extension or external rotation of the thigh during coma or anaesthesia.

Clinical manifestations
- difficulty in flexion of the knee, inability to extend the knee joint
- muscular atrophy of the anterior muscle group of the thigh
- walking with short steps, with the affected leg dragging behind
- inability to run or jump, difficulty in climbing stairs
- hypoaesthesia or anaesthesia at the anterior surface of the thigh and medial surface of the leg and foot and sometimes significant pain at the knee

TREATMENT
Acupoints and techniques

Combination of points	Needles used	Insertion technique	Needling sensation
Biguan (ST-31, affected side)	No. 30 filiform needle, 2 cun in length	Insert towards the medial border of the femur for about 1.8 cun	Local distending pain and/or pain radiating to the knee joint
Jimen (SP-11, affected side)	No. 30 filiform needle, 1.5 cun in length	Insert towards the femur for about 1.0 cun, taking care to avoid damage to the femoral artery and vein, and the saphenous nerve	Local distending pain and/or pain radiating to the medial side of the leg

Xuehai (SP-10, affected side)	No. 30 filiform needle, 2 cun in length	Insert perpendicularly for about 1.5 cun	Local distending pain
Futu (ST-32, affected side)	No. 30 filiform needle, 2 cun in length	Insert towards the medial aspect of the femur for about 1.8 cun	Local distending pain
Yinlingquan (SP-9, affected side)	No. 30 filiform needle, 2 cun in length	Insert perpendicularly towards the fibula for about 1.5 cun	Local distending pain
Heding (EX-LE-2, affected side)	No. 30 filiform needle, 2.5 cun in length	Insert horizontally superiorly towards ST-32 for about 2.3 cun	Local distending pain and/or pain radiating upwards to the inguinal region
Sanyinjiao (SP-6, affected side)	No. 30 filiform needle, 2 cun in length	Insert towards Xuanzhong (GB-39) for 1.0-1.5 cun	Local distending pain

Method
- The patient lies in a supine position.
- The acupoints are needled, with the needles being retained for 40 minutes; during this period, electro-acupuncture is applied.
- Cupping therapy is performed for one minute immediately after the needles are removed.
- Acupuncture should be performed once a day for ten consecutive days (one course of treatment).
- Recommence the treatment after an interval of five days, if necessary.

Clinical notes
This condition is secondary to many other diseases. Electro-acupuncture is applied to treat the condition while the primary disease is being treated. The

therapeutic effects of acupuncture treatment are generally relatively good at the early stage when muscular atrophy is not significant. In cases with muscular atrophy, treatment will take longer to have an effect. The extent to which a cure can be achieved is related to the degree to which the underlying cause is relieved.

45 POLYNEUROPATHY

This is a group of peripheral nervous disorders characterized by simultaneous, usually symmetrical, involvement affecting the distal ends of the limbs more severely than the proximal limbs. The causes are multiple and include nutritional or metabolic impairment, intoxication by heavy metals or industrial chemicals, and post-infectious polyneuritis.

There are no specific pathological changes in this condition. The main changes are non-inflammatory degeneration, presenting segmental demyelination and axon degeneration, with myelin sheath oedema at the early stage, progressing to destruction of the axon.

Clinical manifestations

- symmetrical sensory, motor and autonomic nerve dysfunction, particularly significant at the distal ends of the limbs, with the lower limbs being more affected than the upper limbs
- in cases with sensory impairment, the initially significant symptoms often present as a burning sensation, pain, and paraesthesia or hyperaesthesia, subsequently hypoaesthesia to pain, temperature, touch, vibration and joint position sense
- motor impairments are muscular weakness, paralysis to various degrees, muscular hypotonia, muscular atrophy, and tendon hyporeflexia or areflexia
- autonomic nerve functional impairments are atrophy and tenderness of the skin, hyperkeratosis, sweating, flushing, cyanosis, and a lowering of skin temperature distally in the limbs
- in mild cases, there is only pain and numbness at the distal ends of the limbs without anaesthesia or motor impairment

TREATMENT
Acupoints and techniques

Combination of points	Needles used	Insertion technique	Needling sensation
Waiguan (SJ-5, bilateral)	Two no. 30 filiform needles, 1.5 cun in length	Insert perpendicularly towards Neiguan (PC-6) to a depth of about 1.2 cun, taking care to avoid damage to the median nerve	Local distending pain and/or pain radiating to the dorsum of the hand and the middle finger
Baxie (EX-UE-9, bilateral, eight points in total)	Eight no. 30 filiform needles, 1.5 cun in length	Insert obliquely upwards (at an angle of 45°) along the interosseous metacarpal space for 0.5-1.0 cun	Local distending pain
Sanyinjiao (SP-6, bilateral)	Two no. 30 filiform needles, 2 cun in length	Insert towards Xuanzhong (GB-39) for 1.0-1.5 cun	Local distending pain
Bafeng (EX-LE-10, bilateral, eight points in total)	Eight no. 30 filiform needles, 1.5 cun in length	Insert obliquely upwards (at an angle of 45°) for 0.5-1.0 cun	Local distending pain

Method
- The patient adopts a sitting position.
- The acupoints are needled, with the needles being retained for 40 minutes; during this period, one session of needle rotation is carried out.
- Acupuncture should be performed once a day for ten consecutive days (one course of treatment).
- Recommence the treatment after an interval of five days, if necessary.

Clinical notes

The prognosis for polyneuropathy is good. Generally, when the disease situation is stable (without fever), acupuncture can be performed with relatively good therapeutic results. Clinical experience indicates that acupuncture should not be applied if the body temperature is higher than 38°C. This therapy can shorten the course of the disease and enhance general resistance in combating it. In obstinate cases, the number of local acupoints can be increased. The additional points used depend on the patient's condition; for instance, if it is difficult to stretch the thumb, Shousanli (LI-10) is added; if there is obvious foot-drop, Zusanli (ST-36) and Yanglingquan (GB-34) are added. In cases with muscular atrophy, electro-acupuncture can be employed, although the course of treatment will be longer.

Chapter 4

Other disorders

46 POST-LUMBAR PUNCTURE HEADACHE

Headache after lumbar puncture is caused by leakage of cerebrospinal fluid (CSF) during or after the procedure.

Clinical manifestations
- pain occurs 24-48 hours or later after the procedure
- pain is typically occipital, but may also involve the neck or temporal regions
- pain is aggravated while sitting or standing, and by compressing the carotid vein
- nausea, vomiting, dizziness or visual impairment may occur in some patients

TREATMENT
Acupoints and techniques

Combination of points	Needles used	Insertion technique	Needling sensation
Taiyang (EX-HN-5, bilateral)	Two no. 30 filiform needles, 2 cun in length	Insert horizontally posteriorly towards Shuaigu (GB-8) for 1.0-1.5 cun	Distending pain in the temporal region
Fengchi (GB-20, bilateral)	Two no. 30 filiform needles, 2 cun in length	Insert and push towards the spinal column for 1.0-1.3 cun; as the skin at this location is thick, insertion should be made quickly with the needle then being pushed slowly to the required depth (thus avoiding bending)	Distending pain in the neck and/or pain radiating towards the ipsilateral occiput

Method

- The patient adopts a semi-supine position.
- The acupoints are needled, with the needles being retained for 40 minutes; during this period, one session of needle rotation is carried out.
- Acupuncture should be performed once a day for a maximum of three sessions (see below).

Clinical notes

In most cases, pain can be eliminated after three acupuncture sessions. However, in some cases, the therapeutic effects are not good. In this case, a single dose of extradural corticosteroid injection may be considered. Since injection therapy is invasive and requires extremely skilful placement, it is only indicated when acupuncture has failed after three sessions.

47 **VERTEBRAL ARTERY COMPRESSION SYNDROME**

Vertebral artery compression syndrome is caused by bony encroachment above the level of the 6th cervical vertebra, which compresses the vertebral artery.

Clinical manifestations
- distending pain over the 6th cervical vertebra and instant positional vertigo when the neck is turned 30°-45° in one or both directions depending on whether the bony encroachment is unilateral or bilateral
- lack of sleep, distending pain in the neck, inattention and irritability are the main early symptoms
- development of the disease leads to distending pain in the ocular orbit, visual disturbance, tinnitus, headache, unbearable dizziness when moving the head, nausea and vomiting
- on physical examination, evident tenderness may be found above or below the region of Fengchi (GB-20)
- X-ray may show osteophyte formation or narrowing of the disc space, sometimes with calcification of the ligaments

TREATMENT
Acupoints and techniques

Combination of points	Needles used	Insertion technique	Needling sensation
Fengchi (GB-20, bilateral)	Two no. 30 needles, 2 cun in length	Insert and push towards the spinal column for 1.0-1.3 cun; as the skin at this location is thick, insertion should be made quickly with the needle then being pushed slowly to the required depth (thus avoiding bending)	Distending pain in the neck and/or pain radiating towards the ipsilateral occiput

Fengfu (DU-16)	No. 30 filiform needle, 1 cun in length	Insert perpendicularly to a depth of 0.5-0.8 cun towards the foramen magnum	Distending pain in the occipital region
Taiyang (EX-HN-5, bilateral)	Two no. 30 filiform needles, 2 cun in length	Insert horizontally posteriorly towards GB-8 for 1.0-1.5 cun	Distending pain in the temporal region
Shuaigu (GB-8, bilateral)	Two no. 30 filiform needles, 1.5 cun in length	Insert horizontally posteriorly for about 1.3 cun	Distending pain in the temporal region

Method

- The patient adopts a sitting position.
- The acupoints are needled, with the needles being retained for 40 minutes; during this period, one session of needle rotation with slight stimulation is carried out.
- Acupuncture should be performed once a day for six consecutive days (one course of treatment).
- Recommence the treatment after an interval of three days, if necessary.

Clinical notes

Acupuncture is very effective in the treatment of this disorder. Three to five treatment sessions can basically alleviate the symptoms of vertigo, dizziness, distending headache and distending orbital pain. In severe cases, the symptoms may be attenuated after ten sessions, but relapse usually occurs. After the treatment, the patient should therefore be advised to avoid exposing the neck to cold, to rearrange the pillow frequently and to exercise the neck constantly to strengthen the function of the cervical muscles. Exercise should be by fully flexing the head onto the chest and then hyperextending the neck, followed by lateral flexion of the neck from side to side, trying to approximate the ear to the shoulder; finally, the head should be moved in a circular motion, trying to move the neck through the widest possible range. This sequence should be repeated as often as required. By undertaking these measures, the chances of relapse will be reduced. Prompt treatment of any relapse should ensure rapid recovery.

48 RADICULAR CERVICAL SPONDYLOSIS

Radicular cervical spondylosis results from chronic cervical disc degeneration, with herniation of disc material, secondary calcification, and associated osteophytic outgrowths, causing pressure on nerve roots.

Clinical manifestations

- occurs in both sexes over 35; usually unilateral
- early manifestations are neck pain, limitation of head movement or occipital headache
- radicular pain and other sensory disturbances in the arms and shoulders in some cases
- there may be weakness of the arms
- pain is aggravated when the patient's general health condition is declining (for example, with fever due to cold or inflammation) or inflammatory oedema has developed in the affected part of the cervical vertebrae
- symptoms at the advanced stage include reduction in muscular power, tendon reflexes and skin sensation
- X-rays may show osteophyte formation or narrowing of the disc space, sometimes with calcification of the ligaments

TREATMENT
Acupoints and techniques

Combination of points	Needles used	Insertion technique	Needling sensation
Tianrong (SI-17, affected side)	No. 32 filiform needle, 2 cun in length	Insert under the skin and move the needle slowly in the direction of the transverse process of the 6th cervical vertebra for about 1.6 cun	Pain radiating to the shoulder, arm and hand like an electric shock

Jianzhen (SI-9, affected side)	No. 30 filiform needle, 2 cun in length	Insert perpendicularly towards the inferior part of the shoulder joint for 1.0-1.5 cun	Local distending pain
Tianzong (SI-11, affected side)	No. 30 filiform needle, 2 cun in length	Insert obliquely upwards (at an angle of 45°) for about 1.5 cun	Local distending pain or pain radiating to the upper elbow along the middle of the arm
Jianyu (LI-15, affected side)	No. 30 filiform needle, 2 cun in length	Insert slightly obliquely inferiorly (at an angle of 15° to the skin) towards the elbow for about 1.8 cun	Distending pain in the shoulder or pain radiating down to the upper elbow along the median line of the arm
Shouwuli (LI-13, affected side)	No. 30 filiform needle, 2 cun in length	Insert perpendicularly along the medial border of humerus for 1.0-1.5 cun, taking care to avoid damage to the radial nerve	Local distending pain and/or sensation radiating to the radial side of the wrist
Shousanli (LI-10, affected side)	No. 30 filiform needle, 2 cun in length	Insert perpendicularly to a depth of about 1.5 cun	Local distending pain
Hegu (LI-4, affected side)	No. 30 filiform needle, 2 cun in length	Insert towards Houxi (SI-3) for 1.0-1.5 cun	Distending pain in the palm

Method

- The patient adopts a sitting position.
- The acupoints are needled, with the needles being retained for 40 minutes; during this period, one session of needle rotation with uniform reinforcing-reducing manipulation is carried out.
- Cupping therapy is carried out for one minute immediately after the needles are withdrawn.
- Acupuncture should be performed once a day for ten consecutive days (one course of treatment).
- Recommence the treatment after an interval of five days, if necessary.

Clinical notes

Radicular cervical spondylosis can usually be treated effectively by this therapy if the acupoints are accurately located and the methods followed correctly. Most of the cases with nocturnal aggravation can be effectively alleviated after three treatment sessions. After ten sessions (one course of treatment), the development of pain should be controlled and the pain in the shoulder, arm and hand gradually relieved. Numbness of the hand usually requires a longer course of treatment, which should also bring about a satisfactory result. For the treatment of stubborn cases of longer duration, acupuncture can be combined with other methods of treatment, such as traction or the external application of herbal formulae such as *San Sheng San* (Three-Sage Powder) plus *San Leng* (Rhizoma Sparganii Stoloniferi) and *E Zhu* (Rhizoma Curcumae), which has the function of alleviating pain and transforming blood stasis according to TCM theory.

49 CERVICAL SPONDYLOSIS WITH SYMPATHETIC NERVE INVOLVEMENT

This type of complicated and unpredictable spondylopathy is mainly caused by pressure or stimulation due to strain, trauma, degeneration or hyperplasia of sympathetic nerve fibres. It may lead to a series of symptoms denoting over-activity or underactivity of the sympathetic nerves, usually in association with other types of spondylosis.

Clinical manifestations
- vertigo (irrespective of the position of the neck), heaviness of the head, migraine, occipital or cervical pain
- distending pain in the orbit on the affected side, decrease in visual acuity, ptosis, photophobia, lacrimation
- inattention, fatigue, dilation of the facial vessels on the affected side
- precordial distension or pain in some patients, palpitations, increase in blood pressure, tinnitus
- in some patients, nausea, sensation of a foreign object in the nose, insomnia, cold limbs, constipation and amenorrhoea
- X-ray indicates degeneration of the cervical vertebrae or osteophytosis of the facet joints, and calcification of the ligaments

TREATMENT
Acupoints and techniques

Combination of points	Needles used	Insertion technique	Needling sensation
Fengchi (GB-20, bilateral)	Two no. 30 filiform needles, 2 cun in length	Insert and push towards the spinal column for 1.0-1.3 cun; as the skin at this location is thick, insertion should be made quickly with the needle then being pushed slowly to the required depth (thus avoiding bending)	Distending pain in the neck and/or pain radiating towards the ipsilateral occiput

Jingbailao (EX-HN-15, bilateral)	Two no. 28 filiform needles, 1.5 cun in length	Insert towards the spinal column for 1.0 cun	Distending pain or electric shock-like sensation radiating along the ipsi-lateral forearm and hand
Xueyadian (blood pressure point, bilateral): Located 2 cun lateral to the midpoint between the 6th and 7th cervical vertebrae (see diagram, page 195)	Two no. 30 filiform needles, 2 cun in length	Insert 1.6 cun towards the spinal column	Regional distending pain or pain radiating to the side of the 3rd thoracic vertebra

Method
- The patient adopts a sitting position.
- The acupoints are needled, with the needles being retained for 40 minutes; during this period, one session of needle rotation is carried out.
- After the needles are withdrawn, cupping therapy is performed for one minute.
- Acupuncture should be performed once a day for ten consecutive days (one course of treatment).
- Recommence the treatment after an interval of five days, if necessary.

Clinical notes
The clinical manifestations of this type of spondylopathy are varied, but acupuncture can generally achieve a satisfactory therapeutic effect. If the manifestations are accompanied by symptoms of other types of spondylopathy, treatment can be carried out in accordance with the acupoints selected for the other types.

50 CERVICAL SPONDYLOSIS WITH MYELOPATHY

This spondylopathy is usually caused by pressure on the spinal cord due to encroachment by osteophytic protrusions from the vertebral body, posterior herniation of the intervertebral disc, narrowing of disc space, and calcification of the posterior longitudinal ligament.

Clinical manifestations
- distending pain in the upper limbs, restriction of movement and instability or slight shaking of the entire body when moving or walking
- appropriate treatment at the early stage will prevent lower limb symptoms
- in severe cases, onset of the disease is rapid and usually reaches a peak within one week
- the patient cannot move the neck; even slight movement brings on searing pain in the upper and lower limbs
- sequelae are stiffness of the neck, distending pain in the limbs and diminished motor function
- X-ray shows narrowing of disc space and osteophyte formation, sometimes with calcification of the ligaments
- MRI scan may show disc protrusion

TREATMENT
Acupoints and techniques

Combination of points	Needles used	Insertion technique	Needling sensation
Fengchi (GB-20, bilateral)	Two no. 30 filiform needles, 2 cun in length	Insert and push towards the spinal column for 1.0-1.3 cun; as the skin at this location is thick, insertion should be made quickly with the needle then being pushed slowly to the required depth (thus avoiding bending)	Distending pain in the neck and/or pain radiating towards the ipsilateral occiput

Fengfu (DU-16)	No. 30 filiform needle, 1 cun in length	Insert perpendicularly to a depth of 0.5-0.8 cun towards the foramen magnum	Distending pain in the occipital region
Jingbailao (EX-HN-15, bilateral)	Two no. 28 filiform needles, 1.5 cun in length	Insert towards the spinal column for 1.0 cun	Distending pain or electric shock-like sensation radiating along the ipsilateral forearm and hand
Quchi (LI-11, bilateral)	Two no. 30 filiform needles, 2 cun in length	Insert horizontally and push 1.2-1.5 cun towards Shaohai (HT-3) in the subcutaneous plane	Local distending pain
Jiaji 14th (EX-B-2, bilateral)	Two no. 30 filiform needles, 1 cun in length (no. 28 filiform needles, 1.5 cun in length, can be used for obese patients)	Insert towards the intertransverse muscles of the 2nd and 3rd lumbar vertebrae for about 0.5 cun (0.8 cun for obese patients)	Distending pain or pain radiating to the buttock and lower limb
Huantiao (GB-30, bilateral)	Two no. 28 filiform needles, 4 cun in length	Insert towards the greater sciatic foramen for 3.0-3.5 cun, taking care to avoid damage to the sciatic nerve	Local distending pain or electric shock-like sensation radiating to the ipsilateral lower limb
Scalp acupuncture: Four acupoints in the upper fifth and next two-fifths of the motor and sensory areas	Four no. 30 filiform needles, 1.5 cun in length	Insert for 1.0 cun using the relay puncture technique (see section 19)	Regional distending pain

Method

- The patient lies in a prone position.
- Where one arm is affected, select LI-11 on the affected side.
- Where both arms are affected, select LI-11 on both sides.
- Where the unilateral arm and leg are affected, select LI-11 and GB-30 on the affected side plus the appropriate points in the contralateral motor and sensory areas (see section 19).
- Where all limbs are affected, all the points are selected.
- To treat muscular atrophy, electro-acupuncture is applied to all acupoints except those used for scalp needling.
- The needles in the scalp are manipulated once every 10 minutes.
- Where electro-acupuncture is not used for body acupoints (i.e., when there is no muscular atrophy), the needles are manipulated once every 20 minutes.
- The needles are retained for 40 minutes.
- After the needles are withdrawn, cupping therapy is performed on the body needling points for one minute.
- Acupuncture should be performed once a day for ten consecutive days (one course of treatment).

Clinical notes

In the treatment of pain caused by early cervical spondylosis with myelopathy, needling therapy generally brings quick relief and a satisfactory result. If the curative effect is not satisfactory after 30-60 sessions, it may be necessary to refer for surgical decompression. After the operation, needling therapy can be combined with massage of the upper limbs and hands and functional exercises such as picking up objects, grasping the hand and moving the wrist and arms to improve the strength of the fingers, wrist and arms: the combination of acupuncture, massage and exercises will bring about a satisfactory result.

51 FUNCTIONAL DISORDERS

This term is used to encompass a number of conditions associated with emotional stress or psychological trauma without any organic lesion. Though the clinical features are varied and constitute different entities in a 'Western' medical classification, the acupuncture treatment is identical.

Clinical manifestations

There are four common types:

- aerophagy: the general health of the patient is good; however, there is repeated belching as if the feeling of distension in the stomach was due to the presence of air. After belching, more air is swallowed and the condition is aggravated
- nervous vomiting: often seen in female patients, occurring immediately after eating. Vomiting is continuous and effortless, in small quantities and does not affect intake of food. Usually the patient can continue the meal immediately after vomiting, and experiences no loss of body weight
- anorexia nervosa: the main features are actively maintaining an unduly low weight, morbid concern about weight and body shape, and amenorrhoea in post-pubertal females. Rarely, males may suffer from anorexia nervosa. The patient is extremely emaciated and sometimes exhibits malnutritional oedema. In examining the case history in detail, a predisposing psychological or emotional factor can often be discovered. Patients have an abnormal body image and take steps (including inducing vomiting) to reduce weight. See clinical notes for additional precautions in relation to treatment
- nervous motor impairment: severe pain in the upper abdomen often occurs on an empty stomach due to spasm of the cardiac or pyloric area or the body of the stomach, resulting in difficulty in swallowing and distending pain behind the sternum

TREATMENT
Acupoints and techniques

Combination of points	Needles used	Insertion technique	Needling sensation
Jiuwei (RN-15)	No. 30 filiform needle, 1.5 cun in length	Insert inferiorly at an angle of 25° to the skin for about 1.0 cun, being particularly careful to avoid penetrating the peritoneal cavity in thin subjects	Local distending pain
Zhongwan (RN-12)	No. 30 filiform needle, 1.5 cun in length	Insert perpendicularly for about 1.0 cun, taking care to avoid breaching the peritoneum in very thin subjects	Local distending pain
Zusanli (ST-36, bilateral)	Two no. 30 filiform needles, 2 cun in length	Insert perpendicularly for 1.2-1.5 cun	Local distending pain and/or pain radiating to the dorsum of the foot

Method
- The patient lies in a supine position.
- The acupoints are needled, with the needles being retained for one hour.
- Cupping therapy is performed for about one minute immediately after needle removal.
- Acupuncture should be performed once a day for six consecutive days (one course of treatment).
- Recommence the treatment after an interval of three days, if necessary.

Clinical notes
Acupuncture is relatively effective in the treatment of these functional disorders in the absence of other gastric conditions. The therapeutic effect may be

increased if the doctor can deal with the underlying anxieties and enhance the patient's self-confidence. Bearing in mind the significant morbidity and mortality associated with anorexia nervosa, these patients require skilled psychiatric assessment and support. After recovery, patients should be advised to do more physical exercise to enhance their general constitution and deal with the underlying psychological and emotional problems in order to reduce recurrent conditions.

52 IRRITABLE BOWEL SYNDROME

Irritable bowel syndrome is a condition with functional disturbance of the smooth muscle of the bowel as its main manifestation. It is characterized by intestinal symptoms, such as abdominal discomfort or pain, distension, borborygmi, constipation or diarrhoea.

The pathogenesis of the disease is not completely understood. Three factors may be associated with its pathogenesis – emotional, dietary and altered bowel smooth muscle function.

Clinical manifestations
- recurrent diarrhoea, colic, constipation, or alternating constipation and diarrhoea, excessive mucus in the stool
- in the majority of cases, emotional symptoms also occur, such as dizziness, headache, insomnia, dreaminess, restlessness, emotional instability, irritability, depression, anxiety, low working efficiency, or impaired concentration
- pain in the lower abdomen, especially on the left side
- symptoms may be aggravated under emotional stress, during respiratory infections, or on taking a cold drink
- constipation often occurs in female patients
- the disease is often accompanied by chronic lower abdominal distension, anal fissure, haemorrhoids, abdominal discomfort, tenesmus, halitosis, and dry mouth with a bitter taste
- most patients have functional disturbance of the autonomic nervous system and emotional symptoms, such as profuse sweating, spontaneous perspiration, hot flushes, unstable blood pressure and pulse, a feeling of constriction in the chest, shortness of breath, fatigue, and cold peripheries

Examination
- the percussion note is hyperresonant, and auscultation may reveal increased bowel sounds in the lower central abdomen
- in cases with colic, there may be significant tenderness in the left iliac fossa but no rebound pain, and a prominent colon can be palpated in the area of tenderness
- anal fissure and haemorrhoids can be found in some patients

- insufflation of air during sigmoidoscopy may reproduce the pain of irritable bowel syndrome
- barium enema X-ray may show segmental colonic spasm

TREATMENT
Acupoints and techniques

Combination of points	Needles used	Insertion technique	Needling sensation
Zusanli (ST-36, bilateral)	Two no. 30 filiform needles, 2 cun in length	Insert perpendicularly for 1.2-1.5 cun	Local distending pain and/or pain radiating to the dorsum of the foot
Tianshu (ST-25, bilateral)	Two no. 30 filiform needles, 1.5 cun in length	Insert perpendicularly for about 1.0 cun, taking care to avoid breaching the peritoneum in very thin subjects	Local distending pain
Fujie (SP-14, left side)	No. 30 filiform needle, 1.5 cun in length	Insert perpendicularly for about 1.0 cun, taking care to avoid breaching the peritoneum in very thin subjects	Local distending pain

Method
- The patient lies in a supine position.
- The acupoints are needled, with the needles being retained for 40 minutes; no needle rotation is carried out.
- Cupping therapy is performed for about one minute immediately after needle removal.
- Acupuncture should be performed once a day for ten consecutive days (one course of treatment).
- Recommence the therapy after an interval of five days, if necessary.

Clinical notes

Drug treatment is unsatisfactory in most cases; however, in contrast, acupuncture treatment is relatively effective. Since the disorder can be induced by emotional disturbances, insomnia or too much cold or irritating food, patients should be advised to avoid identifiable precipitating factors, and to review their mental and physical activities; in addition to increasing dietary fibre intake, these are the key points to success.

53 ATYPICAL CHEST PAIN

Atypical chest pain is a symptom with many of the features of cardiac pain but occurring in the absence of any organic cardiac disease. It can be accompanied by other symptoms of anxiety.

Emotional factors such as anxiety, emotional stress, emotional trauma or fatigue play an important role in the aetiology of this disorder and are common predisposing factors. In addition, a lack of physical exercise and poor circulation may mean that a person cannot tolerate even a low level of activity, so a little effort will produce excessive cardiovascular reaction and trigger onset of the condition.

Clinically, the symptoms are quite complicated, and even after improvement, the disease is liable to recur. In a few cases, the course of the disease may last for more than 10 years.

Clinical manifestations
- palpitations: the patient may feel an unduly rapid or irregular heartbeat and precordial pulsation; symptoms may be aggravated after exercise or emotional stress
- precordial pain with no fixed location: the nature of the pain varies; it is most commonly a temporary stabbing pain lasting for a few seconds or a mild, dull pain persisting for several hours
- difficulty in breathing: respiration is often short, shallow and irregular, and accompanied by a sensation of constriction in the chest; it is liable to occur in crowded or poorly ventilated places
- the patient often complains of fatigue, dizziness, insomnia, dream-disturbed sleep or light sleep
- miscellaneous features: the patient is weak, anxious, nervous, depressed or of flat affect, sweats profusely in the palms and armpits, and exhibits a coarse tremor during extension of the fingers

Examination
- brisk tendon reflexes, heart sounds heard easily on auscultation, loud first cardiac sound, tachycardia, occasional ventricular extrasystole
- on X-ray examination, the cardiac size is normal; electrocardiography may show sinus tachycardia

TREATMENT
Acupoints and techniques

Combination of points	Needles used	Insertion technique	Needling sensation
Neiguan (PC-6, bilateral)	Two no. 30 filiform needles, 1.5 cun in length	Insert perpendicularly towards Waiguan (SJ-5) for 1.0-1.3 cun, taking care to avoid damage to the median nerve	Local distending pain and/or pain radiating to the dorsum of the hand and middle finger
Yifeng (SJ-17, bilateral)	Two no. 30 filiform needles, 1.5 cun in length	Insert towards the medial inferior aspect of the mandible for about 1.0 cun	Distending pain in the mandible
Lingxu (KI-24, left side)	No. 30 filiform needle, 1.5 cun in length	Insert horizontally along the intercostal space towards the axilla for about 1.0 cun: great care should be taken to avoid penetrating the pleura	Local distending pain
Shenfeng (KI-23, left side)	No. 30 filiform needle, 1.5 cun in length	Insert horizontally along the intercostal space towards the axilla for about 1.0 cun: great care should be taken to avoid penetrating the pleura	Local distending pain

Method

- The patient lies in a supine position.
- The acupoints are needled, with the needles being retained for 40 minutes.
- Cupping therapy is performed on the two chest points for about one minute immediately after needle removal.
- Acupuncture should be performed once a day for ten consecutive days (one course of treatment).
- Recommence the therapy after an interval of five days, if necessary.

Clinical notes

Acupuncture is very effective in treating cases of cardiac neurosis. The symptoms can generally be eliminated or alleviated after about ten sessions. After recovery, emotional factors may induce recurrence, which can also be treated in the same way. During the intervening period, the patient should be advised to increase physical exercise and to avoid emotional stimulation

54 MYASTHENIA GRAVIS

Myasthenia gravis is a chronic autoimmune disease caused by impairment of acetylcholine transmission at the neuromuscular junctions. This results in characteristic fatiguable skeletal muscle weakness, without pain. The diagnosis is made by the presence of a raised titre of anti-acetylcholine receptor antibody (anti-AchR antibody) or by a positive intravenous edrophonium test.

Myasthenia gravis can present at any age and is sometimes associated with thymic tumour or thyrotoxicosis, rheumatoid arthritis, or disseminated lupus erythematosus. It is more common in women than men.

Clinical manifestations
- onset of the disease can be sudden or insidious
- the disorder is sometimes revealed by the use of muscle relaxants during anaesthesia, concurrent infection or emotional stress; these situations are also associated with an exacerbation of symptoms
- exacerbations may also occur in pregnancy or the postpartum period, or before menstruation

Ocular muscle type
- onset is sudden, presenting usually as diplopia from oculomotor nerve paralysis together with flaccid ptosis of the upper eyelid, hypotropia and exotropia, dilatation of the pupil, and loss of the pupillary light reflex
- after resting, symptoms and signs may improve or disappear. This is the most common type of myasthenia gravis and generally occurs at the early stage

Cervical muscle type
- the lesion involves the trapezius and sternocleidomastoid muscles
- the patient's head is often flexed and needs to be supported due to difficulty in maintaining a 'head-up' posture; impairment makes it impossible to raise the affected arm for a long time, for example for washing the face or combing the hair

Medullary type
- difficulty in chewing and swallowing progressing during the course of a meal, coughing and nasal regurgitation after drinking water, the voice tends to be low with a nasal sound after talking for a time, a 'snarling' smile, hoarse voice and poor enunciation

Systemic type
- onset is slow and progressive and can improve without any intervention

Fulminating type
- in rare cases, onset is sudden and rapidly progresses within a few days or weeks to muscular weakness of the medullary type and respiratory difficulty
- onset can be limited to one type, or aggravated due to infections, emotional stress, fatigue, menstruation, childbirth, or the use of muscle-relaxant anaesthetic agents; it has a tendency to develop into the systemic type in some patients and aggravate rapidly in a short period

TREATMENT
Ocular muscle type
Acupoints and techniques

Combination of points	Needles used	Insertion technique	Needling sensation
Yangbai (GB-14, bilateral)	Two no. 30 filiform needles, 1 cun in length	Insert horizontally inferiorly towards EX-HN-4 for about 0.8 cun	Local distending pain
Cuanzhu (BL-2, bilateral) joining Sizhukong (SJ-23)	Two no. 30 filiform needles, 2 cun in length	Pinch the skin and insert the needle slightly obliquely (at an angle of 15°) at BL-2 for about 0.2 cun and then join SJ-23 horizontally	Distending pain in the orbit
Yuyao (EX-HN-4, bilateral)	Two no. 30 filiform needles, 1 cun in length	Insert along the supra-orbital margin towards the supra-orbital foramen for about 0.5 cun	Distending pain in the orbit
Taiyang (EX-HN-5, bilateral)	Two no. 30 filiform needles, 1 cun in length	Insert at an angle of 25° towards the tip of the ear for about 0.3 cun	Distending pain in the temporal region and/or pain radiating to the medial upper part of the eyeball

Method

- The patient adopts a sitting position.
- The acupoints are needled, with the needles being retained for 40 minutes; during this period, electro-acupuncture is applied.
- Acupuncture should be performed once a day for ten consecutive days (one course of treatment).
- Recommence the therapy after an interval of five days, if necessary.

Systemic type

Acupoints and techniques

The acupoints used for the systemic type are divided into two groups and applied in alternation:

Group 1

Combination of points	Needles used	Insertion technique	Needling sensation
Jiaji (EX-B-2, bilateral)	Two no. 26 filiform needles, 5 cun in length six no. 28 filiform needles, 4 cun in length, and two no. 28 filiform needles, 1 cun in length	See below	Distending pain in the back and waist
Huantiao (GB-30, bilateral)	Two no. 28 filiform needles, 4 cun in length	Insert towards the greater sciatic foramen for 3.0-3.5 cun, taking care to avoid damage to the sciatic nerve	Local distending pain or electric shock-like sensation radiating to the ipsilateral lower limb
Yinmen (BL-37, bilateral)	Two no. 30 filiform needles, 2.5 cun in length	Insert perpendicularly to a depth of about 2.0 cun, taking care to avoid damage to the sciatic nerve	Distending pain in the thigh and/or pain radiating to the lower extremity and foot

Chengshan (BL-57, bilateral)	Two no. 30 filiform needles, 2 cun in length	Insert perpendicularly for 1.0-1.5 cun, taking care to avoid damage to the tibial nerve and popliteal vessels	Local distending pain

Insertion technique for Jiaji points: Starting from Jiaji 1st, the 5 cun needle is inserted horizontally and inferiorly for about 4.8 cun to join Jiaji 5th; the first 4 cun needle is then inserted horizontally at Jiaji 5th to join Jiaji 9th; the second 4 cun needle joins Jiaji 9th to Jiaji 13th; the third 4 cun needle joins Jiaji 13th to Jiaji 17th; the 1 cun needle is inserted perpendicularly at Jiaji 17th for 0.3-0.5 cun. The manoeuvre is the same on both sides

Method
- The patient lies in a prone position.
- The acupoints are needled, with the needles being retained for 40 minutes; during this period, electro-acupuncture is applied.
- Cupping therapy is applied for about one minute immediately after needle removal.
- Acupuncture should be performed every other day alternating with the points in group 2 for 20 consecutive sessions (one course of treatment).
- Recommence the treatment after an interval of five days, if necessary.

Group 2

Combination of points	Needles used	Insertion technique	Needling sensation
Tianding (LI-17, bilateral)	Two no. 30 filiform needles, 1 cun in length	Insert towards the spinal column for about 0.5 cun, taking care to avoid damage to the external jugular vein and supra-clavicular nerves	Local distending pain and/or pain radiating to the upper arm and hand

Hegu (LI-4, bilateral)	Two no. 30 filiform needles, 2 cun in length	Insert towards Houxi (SI-3) for 1.0-1.5 cun	Distending pain in the palm
Qianzheng (bilateral): Located 0.5 cun anterior to and level with the medial point of the ear lobe (see diagram, page 195)	Two no. 30 filiform needles, 2 cun in length	Insert slightly obliquely (at an angle of 15°) for about 1.3 cun towards the apex of the nose; in order to avoid injury to the parotid gland and the mandibular vessels, do not puncture too deeply	Local distending pain and heavy sensation
Shangwan (RN-13)	No. 28 filiform needle, 4 cun in length	Insert slightly obliquely (at an angle of 15° to the skin surface) towards Shenque (RN-8) for about 3.8 cun	Local distending pain
Zusanli (ST-36, bilateral)	Two no. 30 filiform needles, 2 cun in length	Insert perpendicularly for 1.2-1.5 cun	Local distending pain and/or pain radiating to the dorsum of the foot
Sanyinjiao (SP-6, bilateral)	Two no. 30 filiform needles, 2 cun in length	Insert towards Xuanzhong (GB-39) for 1.0-1.5 cun	Local distending pain

Method
- The patient lies in a supine position.
- The acupoints are needled, with the needles being retained for 40 minutes; during this period, electro-acupuncture is applied.

- Cupping therapy is applied at LI-17, RN-13, ST-36 and SP-6 for about one minute immediately after needle removal.
- Acupuncture should be performed every other day alternating with the points in group 1 for 20 consecutive sessions (one course of treatment).
- Recommence the treatment after an interval of five days, if necessary.

Clinical notes

Myasthenia gravis is a condition which may not respond well to drug treatment. The therapeutic effect of electro-acupuncture for the treatment of the ocular muscle type is relatively good; the therapy has some effect on other types. Where it is ineffective, oral pyridostigmine therapy during acupuncture gives better results than where pyridostigmine is used alone. Ocular symptoms which respond incompletely to pyridostigmine usually improve with prednisolone therapy. Patients with serious manifestations (such as weakness of the respiratory muscle, dyspnoea or swallowing difficulties) should be hospitalized and acupuncture can be used as an accessory treatment. The two groups of acupuncture points for the systemic type are used alternately; this has a certain therapeutic effect in strengthening the respiratory muscle and other muscles throughout the body. Cases associated with thymoma require surgical management because of the risk of local spread: however, the symptoms of myasthenia rarely improve after surgery. Since myasthenia gravis is a complex condition with a variety of symptoms and signs, the acupoints listed above should be modified in accordance with the variations encountered.

55 PERIODIC PARALYSIS

Periodic paralysis is a group of diseases characterized by recurrences of flaccid paralysis of the skeletal muscles. The disease is divided into three types depending on the potassium level in the blood at the time of the attack – hyperkalaemic, hypokalaemic and normokalaemic. Hypokalaemic periodic paralysis is the most common type; it is often misdiagnosed as cerebrovascular disease or cerebral paralysis on first presentation. Serum potassium determination during the attack and electrocardiogram examinations can confirm the diagnosis.

Clinical manifestations
The clinical manifestations of the three types are as follows:
Hypokalaemic periodic paralysis
- mainly occurs in young people, more likely to affect males than females; typically, attacks occur at night
- the patient feels paralysis (usually symmetrical) of the limbs after waking
- the attack may also start from the lower limbs and spread to the upper limbs, with the proximal parts of the limbs being more severely affected; trunk muscles may also be involved
- in some severe cases, respiration and swallowing can be affected
- sometimes eyelid ptosis occurs, but extraocular muscles are rarely paralysed
- tone of the affected muscles is lowered, tendon reflexes may be decreased or absent, and response to mechanical or electrical stimulus is weakened and may even disappear
- in severe cases with recurrent attack, weakness and atrophy may develop in the muscles at the proximal end of the lower limbs, in front of the tibia and in the back
- prodromal symptoms include ache or distension, numbness in the limbs, thirst, sweating, oliguria, flushes and fright
- during the prodromal or early paralytic stage, moving the involved limbs may inhibit the attack. The earliest paralysed muscle will be restored first. Sweating may often accompany the restoration, and some patients may feel that the involved muscles are stiff and painful after muscular strength is restored
- the serum potassium level falls during an attack, but may not actually drop below the normal range
- electromyography shows that the excitement threshold is elevated in mild cases, and disappears in severe cases

Hyperkalaemic periodic paralysis

- during the onset of symptoms, the serum potassium level rises, but this may be only a slight change
- the disease is aggravated by potassium loading or ameliorated by sodium loading
- the attack has no predilection for either sex, usually begins before 10 years of age, and occurs in the daytime; in severe cases, it takes place several times a day for short periods, dozens of minutes to several hours, or occasionally for more than two days
- precipitating factors include resting after vigorous exercise, emotional stress, cold, hunger, pregnancy, alcohol intake, infection and general anaesthesia
- the symptoms and signs of the attack are similar to but may be milder than for the hypokalaemic type. Occasionally, arrhythmia such as bigeminy or paroxysmal tachycardia may be found

Normokalaemic periodic paralysis

- the attack often occurs before 10 years of age, and frequently begins at night or early in the morning. During the attack, part or all of the limb muscles are paralysed
- the attack lasts for a relatively long time, several days to several weeks
- rest after physical exercise may precipitate the attack
- some patients are fond of salty food; decrease of salt intake or substitution with potassium salt may precipitate or aggravate the symptoms
- during the onset of paralysis, the potassium levels in the serum and urine are normal

TREATMENT
Acupoints and techniques

Combination of points	Needles used	Insertion technique	Needling sensation
Tianding (LI-17, bilateral)	Two no. 30 filiform needles, 1 cun in length	Insert towards the spinal column for about 0.5 cun, taking care to avoid damage to the external jugular vein and supra-clavicular nerves	Local distending pain and/or pain radiating to the upper arm and hand

Quchi (LI-11, bilateral)	Two no. 30 filiform needles, 2 cun in length	Insert perpendicularly for about 1.5 cun, taking care to avoid damage to the radial nerve	Local distending pain
Hegu (LI-4, bilateral)	Two no. 30 filiform needles, 2 cun in length	Insert towards Houxi (SI-3) for 1.0-1.5 cun	Distending pain in the palm
Futu (ST-32, bilateral)	Two no. 30 filiform needles, 2.5 cun in length	Insert obliquely upwards (at an angle of 45°) for about 2.0 cun	Local distending pain
Zusanli (ST 36, bilateral)	Two no. 30 filiform needles, 2 cun in length	Insert perpendicularly for 1.2-1.5 cun	Local distending pain and/or pain radiating to the dorsum of the foot
Neiting (ST-44, bilateral)	Two no. 30 filiform needles, 1.5 cun in length	Insert obliquely upwards (at an angle of 45°) for about 1.0 cun	Local distending pain

Method

- The patient lies in a supine position.
- The acupoints are needled, with the needles being retained for 40 minutes; during this period, electro-acupuncture is applied.
- Cupping therapy is applied at LI-17, LI-11, ST-32 and ST-36 for about one minute immediately after needle removal.
- Acupuncture should be performed once a day for ten consecutive days (one course of treatment).
- Recommence the treatment after an interval of five days, if necessary.

Clinical notes

The disease is often self-limiting. Acupuncture can shorten the duration of the disease and enhance the patient's general resistance. For chronic cases with partial muscular atrophy, the points listed above should be expanded and modified to adapt to the conditions encountered. For instance, if there is atrophy of the thenar, hypothenar and lumbrical muscles, Baxie (EX-UE-9) on the affected side or both sides can be added; if there is myophagism of the dorsum of the foot, Bafeng (EX-LE-10) on the affected side or both sides can be added. Although the treatment period is relatively long (30-60 sessions), satisfactory therapeutic effects can be obtained.

56 **PHANTOM LIMB PAIN**

Phantom limb pain refers to a pain sensation felt as if an amputated limb were still present.

Clinical manifestations
- phantom limb pain often occurs after amputation (in most instances affecting the lower limb) after the surface of the wound has healed
- in the majority of cases, the pain occurs at night and may wake the patient
- after waking, the patient may perceive pain for several hours or days, and feel as if the amputated extremity still exists
- the pain is severe, lancinating or searing in nature, and may persist with paroxysmal aggravation

TREATMENT
Acupoints and techniques

Combination of points	Needles used	Insertion technique	Needling sensation
Baihui (DU-20)	No. 30 filiform needle, 1 cun in length	Insert slightly obliquely postero-inferiorly (at an angle of 15°) towards Houding (DU-19) for about 0.5 cun	Local distending pain
Hegu (LI-4, bilateral)	Two no. 30 filiform needles, 2 cun in length	Insert towards Houxi (SI-3) for 1.0-1.5 cun	Distending pain in the palm
Zusanli (ST-36, unaffected side)	No. 30 filiform needle, 2 cun in length	Insert perpendicularly for 1.2-1.5 cun	Local distending pain and/or pain radiating to the dorsum of the foot

Method
- The patient lies in a supine position.
- The acupoints are needled, with the needles being retained for 40 minutes; during this period, one session of needle rotation is carried out.
- Acupuncture should be performed once a day until the pain is eliminated.

Clinical notes
The therapeutic effects of acupuncture in phantom limb pain are relatively good. Rotation manipulation should be vigorous; the more vigorous the manipulation, the better the therapeutic results. Strong stimulation can control the pain in most cases, but it may recur several hours after alleviation. If acupuncture treatment is applied daily, the symptoms will be gradually relieved.

57 TRAUMATIC PARAPLEGIA

Paraplegia is caused by trauma of the spinal cord and can be divided into quadriplegia (paralysis of all limbs due to cervical cord damage) and paraplegia (paralysis of both legs due to damage to the thoracic or lumbar cord).

Paraplegia often complicates injuries of the thoracic or lumbar spine. The types of injury most likely to result in paraplegia from spinal cord damage are 'burst' fractures and fracture dislocations of the thoracolumbar region.

Clinical manifestations

- following cord damage there is complete paralysis and anaesthesia with loss of the anal reflex ('spinal shock'); if the anal reflex returns and the neurological deficit persists, this is a diagnostic of complete cord transection
- in incomplete cord damage, spinal shock may only last for a short time, generally less than 24-48 hours
- after recovery from spinal shock, flaccid paralysis may occur below the transverse damage
- if the spinal cord is not injured or compressed, rapid recovery can be expected
- where there is severe spinal cord trauma, atrophy may occur in the muscles of the lower extremities, which may be flaccid initially, gradually becoming atrophic

TREATMENT
Acupoints and techniques

Combination of points	Needles used	Insertion technique	Needling sensation
Shenshu (BL-23, bilateral)	Two no. 28 filiform needles, 2 cun in length	Insert towards the intertransverse space of the 1st and 2nd lumbar vertebrae for 1.0-1.5 cun	Numbness and distending pain radiating to the ipsilateral leg

Dachangshu (BL-25, bilateral)	Two no. 30 filiform needles, 2 cun in length	Insert towards the bony surface of the transverse process of the 5th lumbar vertebra for about 1.5 cun	Local distending pain and/or pain radiating to the lower extremity
Huantiao (GB-30, bilateral)	Two no. 28 filiform needles, 4 cun in length	Insert towards the greater sciatic foramen for 3.0-3.5 cun, taking care to avoid damage to the sciatic nerve	Local distending pain or electric shock-like sensation radiating to the ipsilateral lower limb
Yinmen (BL-37, bilateral)	Two no. 30 filiform needles, 2.5 cun in length	Insert perpendicularly to a depth of about 2.0 cun, taking care to avoid damage to the sciatic nerve	Distending pain in the thigh and/or pain radiating to the lower extremity and foot
Weizhong (BL-40, bilateral)	Two no. 30 filiform needles, 1.5 cun in length	Insert slightly obliquely upwards (at an angle of 15°) for about 1.0 cun, taking care to avoid damage to the tibial nerve and popliteal vessels	Distending pain in the popliteal fossa
Chengshan (BL-57, bilateral)	Two no. 30 filiform needles, 2 cun in length	Insert perpendicularly for 1.0-1.5 cun, taking care to avoid damage to the tibial nerve and popliteal vessels	Local distending pain

Method

- The patient lies in a prone position.
- The acupoints are needled, with the needles being retained for 40 minutes; during this period, electro-acupuncture is applied.
- Cupping therapy is applied for about one minute immediately after needle removal.
- Acupuncture should be performed once a day for ten consecutive days (one course of treatment).
- Recommence the treatment after an interval of five days, if necessary.

Clinical notes

Acupuncture is effective in treating paraplegia and is primarily indicated for mild paraplegia caused by compression, or where compression has been relieved by earlier surgical management while the spinal cord itself is intact. Where there is severe or complete spinal cord damage, or compression has not been relieved, the treatment can only temporarily (for instance, after 30 treatment sessions and for 15-30 days after acupuncture treatment is ended) restore partial muscular tone, part of the atrophic muscles, or part of any nerves not seriously damaged. When acupuncture is terminated, the pre-treatment situation may recur or the involved muscles become atrophic again. The effect depends primarily on the degree of damage in the spinal cord and the extent to which compression is relieved.

Where there is fracture, fracture-dislocation or compression by bone fragments, surgery should be performed as early as possible to reduce the fractured bone(s) or remove the bone fragments. Post-operation paraplegia may be similar to that before the operation, i.e. paraplegia below the damaged vertebra(e) and spinal cord segment. The involved muscles may be flaccid or completely spastic. Acupuncture may help in recovery if the damage is not very severe or the compression by haematoma or fracture is of short duration and a successful operation has been performed at an early stage.

Appendix: Location of acupuncture points referred to in the book

Lung Meridian, LU   182
LU-2   Yunmen
LU-10   Yuji

Large Intestine Meridian, LI   183
LI-4   Hegu
LI-10   Shousanli
LI-11   Quchi
LI-13   Shouwuli
LI-14   Binao
LI-15   Jianyu
LI-16   Jugu
LI-17   Tianding
LI-20   Yingxiang

Stomach Meridian, ST   184
ST-1   Chengqi
ST-2   Sibai
ST-4   Dicang
ST-6   Jiache
ST-7   Xiaguan
ST-8   Touwei
ST-9   Renying
ST-25   Tianshu
ST-31   Biguan
ST-32   Futu
ST-36   Zusanli
ST-44   Neiting

Spleen Meridian, SP   185
SP-6   Sanyinjiao
SP-9   Yinlingquan
SP-10   Xuehai

SP-11   Jimen
SP-14   Fujie

Heart Meridian, HT   186
HT-3   Shaohai
HT-7   Shenmen

Small Intestine Meridian, SI   187
SI-3   Houxi
SI-9   Jianzhen
SI-11   Tianzong
SI-17   Tianrong

Bladder Meridian, BL   188
BL-1   Jingming
BL-2   Cuanzhu
BL-10   Tianzhu
BL-11   Dazhu
BL-23   Shenshu
BL-24   Qihaishu
BL-25   Dachangshu
BL-37   Yinmen
BL-40   Weizhong
BL-54   Zhibian
BL-57   Chengshan
BL-60   Kunlun

Kidney Meridian, KI   189
KI-23   Shenfeng
KI-24   Lingxu

Pericardium Meridian, PC   189
PC-2   Tianquan
PC-6   Neiguan

Scalp acupuncture
Balance area   202
Chorea and tremor area   201
Foot motor and sensory area   202
Motor area   200, 201

Praxis area   201
Sensory area   201
Speech area no. 2   201, 202
Speech area no. 3   201
Vasomotor area   201

Note: In some of the diagrams in the following pages, certain points additional to those of the relevant meridian have been included in order to facilitate identification and location.

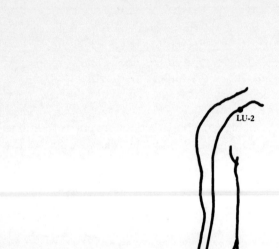

Points of Lung Meridian, LU

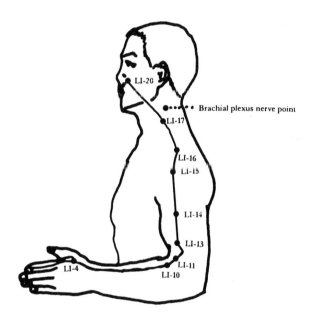

Points of Large Intestine Meridian, LI

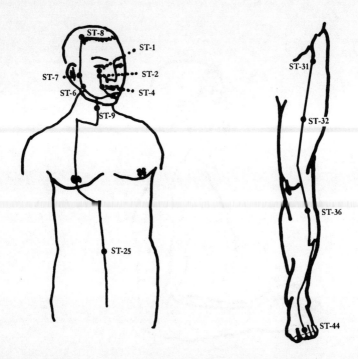

Points of Stomach Meridian, ST

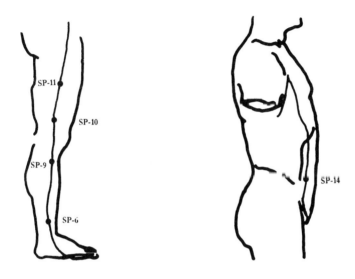

Points of Spleen Meridian, SP

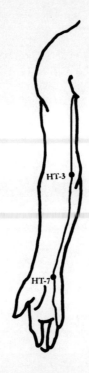

Points of Heart Meridian, HT

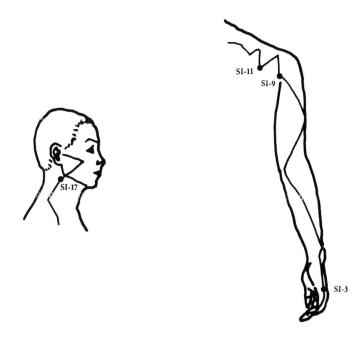

Points of Small Intestine Meridian, SI

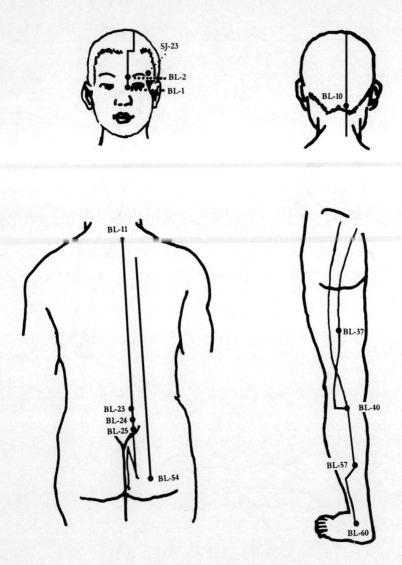

Points of Bladder Meridian, BL

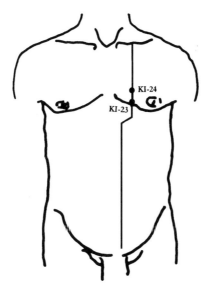

Points of Kidney Meridian, KI

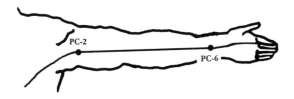

Points of Pericardium Meridian, PC

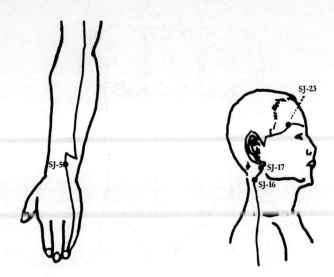

Points of Sanjiao Meridian, SJ

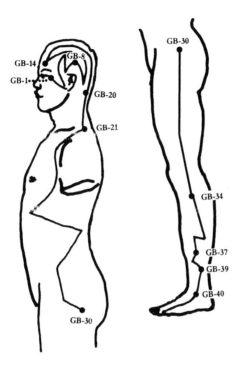

Points of Gallbladder Meridian, GB

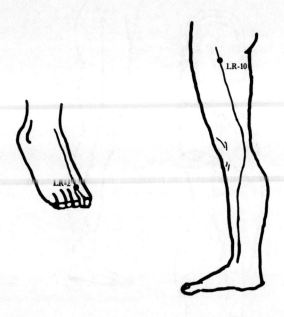

Points of Liver Meridian, LR

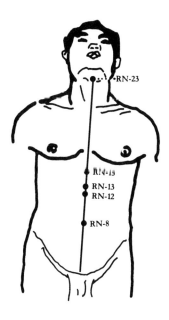

Points of Ren (Conception Vessel) Meridian, RN

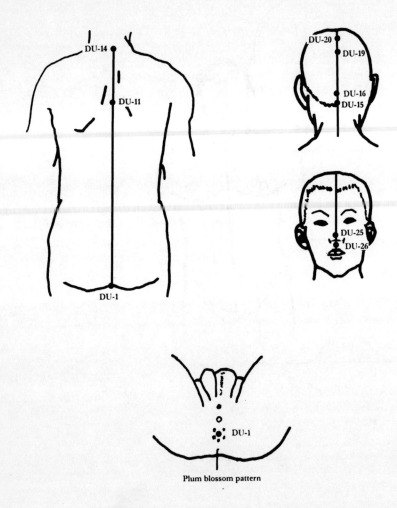

Points of Du (Governor Vessel) Meridian, DU

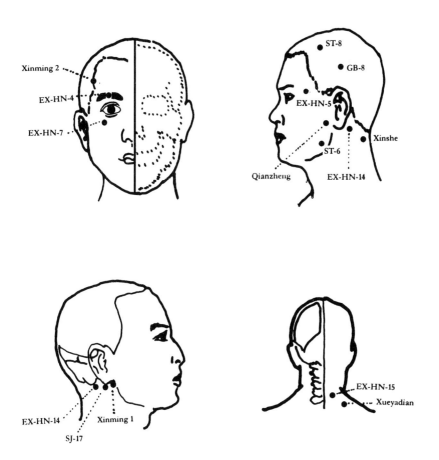

Extra Points
Head and Neck, EX-HN

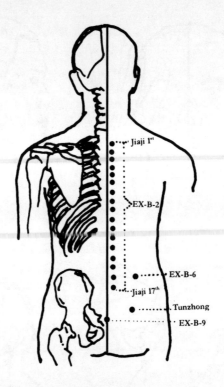

Extra Points
Back, EX-B

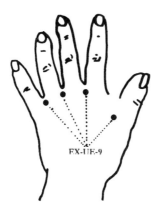

EX-UE-9

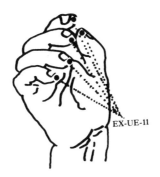

EX-UE-11

Extra Points
Upper Extremities, EX-UE

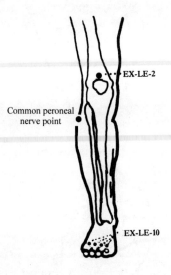

Extra Points
Lower Extremities, EX-LE

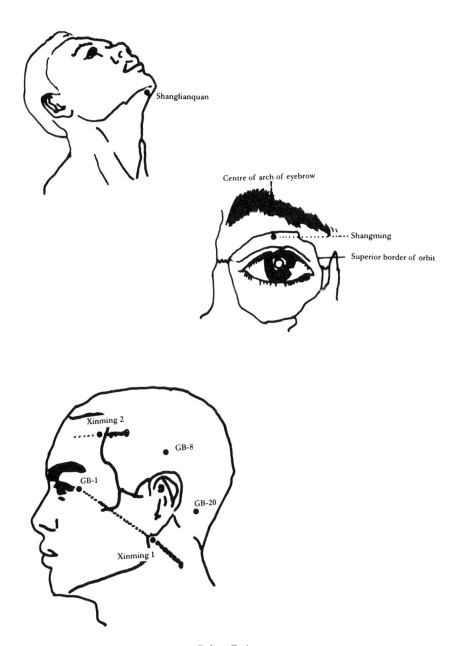

Shanglianquan

Centre of arch of eyebrow

Shangming

Superior border of orbit

Xinming 2

GB-8

GB-1

GB-20

Xinming 1

Other Points

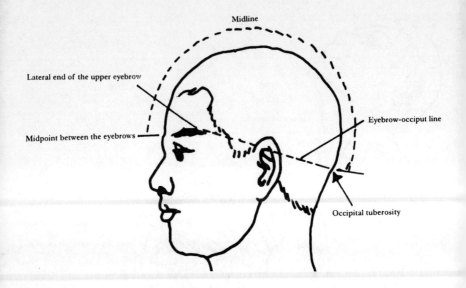

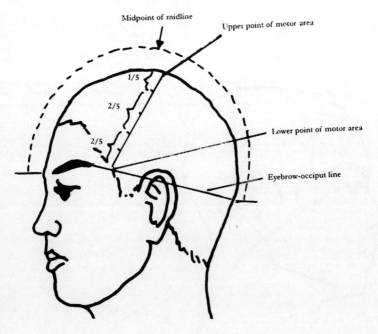

Scalp Acupuncture

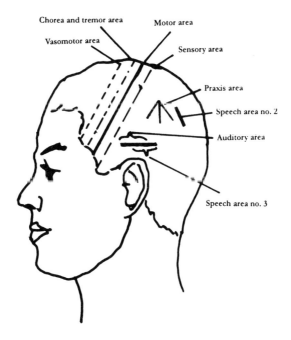

Scalp Acupuncture

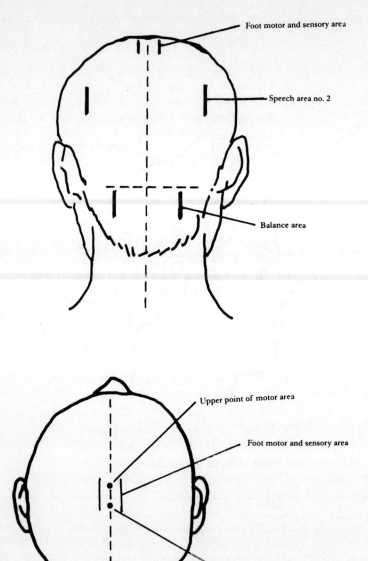

Scalp Acupuncture

Bibliography

Chinese Academy of Traditional Chinese Medicine, *Atlas of Standard Acupuncture Points*, Qingdao: Qingdao Publishing House, 1991.

Henan Journal of New Medicine (compilers), *Foundations of Medicine: The Nervous System*, Beijing: People's Medical Publishing House, 1977.

Du Naiqiang, *Integrated Chinese and Western Medicine Used in the Treatment of Cardiovascular and Cerebrovascular Diseases*, Taiyuan: Shanxi Higher University Joint Publishing House, 1992.

Fu Qiang, *A Comprehensive Clinical Guide to Practical Acupuncture Treatment*, Beijing: Traditional Chinese Medicine and Pharmacology Publishing House, 1991.

Liang Hongzhi, *Emergency Treatment of Cardiovascular and Cerebrovascular Diseases*, Tianjin: Tianjin Science and Technology Translation Publishing Company, 1994.

Lu Shoukang, *Complete Practical Scalp Acupuncture*, Shanghai: Shanghai Science and Technology Publishing House, 1993.

Shandong Medical College Compiling Group, *Human Morphology*, Beijing: People's Medical Publishing House, 1976.

State Bureau of Technical Supervision of the People's Republic of China, *The National Standard of the People's Republic of China: Location of Points*, Beijing: State Bureau of Technical Supervision, 1990.

Wang Xiaozhong, *Disorders of the Nervous System*, Beijing: People's Medical Publishing House, 1979.

Wang Xuetai, *Complete Chinese Acupuncture*, Zhengzhou: Henan Science and Technology Publishing House, 1992.

Xiang Jiarong, *Practical Neurology*, Tianjin: Tianjin Science and Technology Translation Publishing Company, 1992.

Zhao Junli, *Cardiovascular and Cerebrovascular Diseases*, Tianjin: Tianjin Science and Technology Translation Publishing Company, 1992.

Zhou Deyu, *Human Anatomy*, Changsha: Hunan Science and Technology Publishing House, 1991.

Index